Laura Mansell holds a first class honours degree and post-graduate diploma in adult nursing, and has additional qualifications in neuro-linguistic programming and life coaching. Using reflections of her own childhood and subsequent adulthood abuse, trauma and the effects of this on her mental and physical health, she aims to analyse toxic behavioural patterns and use the word of God and prayer as a powerful tool for healing.

To my Mum: Thank you for everything. I love you always.

To my Brothers: Proverbs 17:17. Thank you for always protecting, supporting and believing in me.

To Melody: My Sister, My Friend. My inspiration. A light in the darkness.

Laura Mansell

BREAKING CHAINS – 'THE WORD'

AUSTIN MACAULEY PUBLISHERS™
LONDON · CAMBRIDGE · NEW YORK · SHARJAH

Copyright © Laura Mansell 2023

The right of Laura Mansell to be identified as the author of this work has been asserted by the author in accordance with sections 77 and 78 of the Copyright, Designs and Patents Act 1988.

All rights reserved. No part of this publication may be reproduced, stored in a retrieval system, or transmitted in any form or by any means, electronic, mechanical, photocopying, recording, or otherwise, without the prior permission of the publishers.

Any person who commits any unauthorised act in relation to this publication may be liable to criminal prosecution and civil claims for damages.

All of the events in this memoir are true to the best of author's memory. The views expressed in this memoir are solely those of the author.

A CIP catalogue record for this title is available from the British Library.

ISBN 9781035812752 (Paperback)
ISBN 9781035812769 (ePub e-book)

www.austinmacauley.com

First Published 2023
Austin Macauley Publishers Ltd®
1 Canada Square
Canary Wharf
London
E14 5AA

Table of Contents

Backstory	9
Setting the Scene	13
Childhood Abuse and Its Links to Mental Health	25
Toxic Relationships	39
Personality Disorders	56
Psychology	63
Analysing	72
Victimhood	76
Self-Hate – Self Love (The In-between)	81
Who Are You?	85
Losing What No Longer Serves You	91
It's a Choice	96
Empathy	99
Compassion and Conscience	103
Mindfulness and NLP	106
Present vs Preoccupied	117

Finding Your Purpose	**122**
Prayers that Break Chains	**126**
Conclusion	**130**
References	**132**

Backstory

Isaiah 48:10: "Behold, I have refined you, but not with silver; I have tested you in the furnace of affliction."

It has been a good while since I attended church. The last time I encountered the pure, unreversed love of my creator in the presence of his faithful followers was back in or around the millennium.

I gave my life to God at the age of 11. I had always known that there was more to my existence, my thoughts, my feelings and my uniqueness than a simple explosion of matter.

My God is an awesome God.

I trundled through life and faith for a number of years. Growing up surrounded by friends and acquaintances who went to church, sang the hymns, listened to the message and then lived by their own rules once the doors closed at the end of the service.

I always remember feeling that God was real but never actually knew His mightiness. I understood that he was omnipresent but never really experienced the power of his companionship. It took a great deal of time to realise that he has always been with me, even when I turned away from his face by way of my own sinful living.

Whilst attending church, around the age of 15, God spoke to me through a prophet about becoming a nurse and visiting Uganda. I began studying for a diploma in Nursing a few years later, at 17 and a half. During this time, I began falling away from the church. Partly due to my own teenage rebellion, and partly due to the insidious false nature of some members and leaders of the congregation.

I was never swayed by what people would consider a 'big sin'. I was never an evil person, never went out of my way to hurt anyone (not purposefully anyway), never stole, and never acted in a way whereby others would suffer. However, I wasn't a woman of God either. Not by a long shot.

Instead of concentrating on achieving my diploma and becoming a nurse, I stayed out late, drank too much, spent all of my money on things I didn't need, meddled in smoking weed and generally stopped focusing on the right things. I also declared that I wasn't 'good enough' to pass the assignments I was given, deciding I wasn't academic enough to get the required marks. I declared this out loud to whoever would listen. It wasn't true, but it manifested.

After 7 months, and a few failed assignments, I gave up. I stepped away from the course, stepped away from the church, from God and stepped into a relationship with an ungodly partner. Years rolled by, men came and went, others I left before things got 'serious', jobs came and went, money was earned and spent, and nothing seemed to stick.

Fast forward to six years ago. I started working for a local college. One of four staff members who were selected to support the young people with gaining employment. The company, however, similar to others in this sector, were more concerned with targets and earnings than touching and changing people's lives on a deeper level. I'm not sure if this was the first time, I had thought this thought but I remember it deeply troubling my spirit. It's hard to define how you suddenly, after years of witnessing what we will discuss later as toxic and unfulfilling people, places and things, feel a shift that begins an epiphany in your soul.

As it happened that day, one of the four selected new-employees didn't turn up for their position, and in stepped Melody.

God is good and has a plan. I was right where he wanted me to be. Back on his path.

Whether these words echo off the page for you right now, or you look at them quizzically and wonder if I've lost my mind, all I can say is that if you trust, believe and look for God's little synchronicities or acts of divine intervention in your life, you will absolutely see them.

Melody and I had an instant connection. Only God will put people like her in your midst. We soon realised that we were in the presence of two colleagues who were somewhat emotionally challenged, and possibly one of whom had distinct narcissistic tendencies or traits of a similar personality disorder. It was here that we would later learn that God was beginning to uncover a specific set of circumstances in both of our lives which would come full circle into the present-day ministering of his work.

The short amount of time we spent together in that workplace built a truly strong friendship and a foundation of what we believe is our calling. Both Melody and I went through some of the hardest moments of our lives together. Like rocks, we carried each other. We also realised that we had very similar backstories, with familial issues encompassing similar behavioural patterns, similar traits in us because of them and a yearning to learn as much as we could about psychology, health, education, well-being and, at the centre of it all, God.

Melody will tell her own story in her own way if she feels she is called to do so, and here within this book, I will tell you mine.

Setting the Scene

1 Timothy 4:12: "Don't let anyone look down on you because you are young, but set an example for the believers in speech, in life, in love, in faith and in purity."

My mum became very ill during the initial period of my friendship with Melody. She was diagnosed with cancer, given a one in twenty chance of survival and only IF they did a very intrusive surgery on her to remove part of her pancreas, stomach and liver.

I recall the day Mum was in surgery for ten hours and I had a heavy burden on my heart. I might lose my best friend. Melody supported me without hesitating, even through her own anguish and personal struggles during the same time, with prayer and understanding, warmth and love, she supported me and gave strength through her knowledge of the Word of God.

Mum pulled through the operation, and the next few weeks were a blur. Visiting her in intensive care every night, often straight from work where pressure was building to perform and earn the company money whilst fighting some kind of spiritual battle with the energies surrounding me in that space. All I had to offer was my presence. My strength of character, my vision, my kindness, my work ethic, my love – it seemed none of those traits were required, and if anything were frowned upon like some stumbling block to a team more interested in figures and number crunching than in actual people.

My heart was in the hospital. My mind was questioning why people were so cruel and uninterested in the things that actually matter, in relationships and belonging and most of all, in love.

Being on the ward each night led me to question my decision to quit nursing. Seeing angels in scrubs taking care of my loved one, my mother, in the most gracious, perfectly imperfect way, with a serving and giving spirit, with empathy and kindness.

Why did I ever turn my back on my calling?

Fast forward a few weeks later and Mum pulled through. It just-so-happened that the cancer was in 'exactly' the right position in her bile duct to have blocked it off, producing the symptoms that led to identifying it early enough to ensure it could be removed successfully, with no lymph node involvement. The cancer hadn't spread and the tumour was removed. It was by the Lord's amazing grace that Mum survived. And by His mighty plan, I followed my path because of this. A crisis proceeding to a victory. It's difficult to see the plans the Lord has for us when it all seems dark and grey and like life is giving us a hard time, but Jesus knows. He always knows.

I recall being back in the office soon after this, pondering the thought of returning to study. I looked online, saw that my town's very own university had a nursing degree course starting the month after, and applied there and then. It was as if I couldn't wait another minute.

I don't know what I expected to happen, but I almost felt as if I rushed the application so much that I didn't stand a chance. It was almost as if I'd done the whole thing on a whim or somewhat unconsciously.

I spoke to Melody about it in an almost blasé manner, 'what will be will be'. I think that Melody realised that it was, in fact, a call from God.

A week later, I received an email inviting me for an interview.

A week after that, whilst running an event at the college, I received confirmation that I had a place on the course.

I remember being so excited that I literally ran into the room where we were delivering sessions to the students and squealed with delight at Melody at the prospect of leaving that awful job and doing something I felt my heart longed for! My purpose.

Two weeks later, I sat in a new classroom, with a new group of friends, starting a new chapter.

The three years I spent doing that degree were some of the toughest, and yet blessed years of my life. I relied on so many people for so much and yet found my own strength in realising that 'I am good enough', through focus, education, developing my strengths and working on my limitations.

I studied, I learnt and I gratefully received support from others, financially, spiritually and emotionally. I attended every single day I was expected to attend and fought to get my qualification.

During year two of the course, I began to get back pain. Annoying at first but then limiting and excruciating to the point where I couldn't stand up for more than 20 minutes without being in agony.

Not ideal when placements expected you to be on your feet for 12 and a half hours at a time. I ended up having back surgery and six weeks off in my second year.

University wasn't particularly supportive during this time, with the main consensus being that I would simply have to drop out of study for six months in order to heal and then return with the cohort behind me, to finish up.

Instead, I fought to stay put and finally won. This must have only been possible by the grace of God upon my life and his promise, being yes and amen.

I got over surgery and carried on through year two and into year three. During those years, I also fought a battle with my weight. I had always been 'larger than average' and put it down to genetics. All the ladies in my family are of 'big build'. My weight however had nothing to do with being this way. I had eaten my way to 19 stone.

The reason for this, I later acknowledged, lay deeply rooted in my own childhood abuse.

I ate for comfort.

I ate to make myself feel like the unattractive person I wanted to be, to stop admiring glances from men who were 'all the same'.

I ate to disassociate myself from sexualisation.

I ate to make myself feel better.

I will cover this more in a separate chapter, but the importance of telling this now is that I fought the battle with my weight during these years too.

By year three of my course, I was 13 stone. 1 stone to go until I reached a healthy target for my height.

I began to pray during this time to meet a man. There's such an expectation on women, even now in the twenty-first century, to get married, to settle down and to be loved and looked after by a man, to have children and to rely on one another for strength and support. Whilst I don't entirely disagree that the right relationship can provide a strong foundation and rock for many, I also see all too well how the wrong relationship can impact you in ways that are unacceptable and, for want of a better phrase, soul-destroying. I see this too often and it breaks my heart. But back then, before the journey I've since endured, I wanted to be accepted and to be one of the women who fulfilled the expectation of having a husband and children, the perfect family and a white picket fence. It's only now, with hindsight being 20-20, that I see the mirage in many, many perfect family photos.

I put my trust in God for the first time in years to find me a man! The God who I'd turned away from for such a long time was now being asked to find me a man who would love me unconditionally. Who would see my struggles and battles and see that I'd overcome them and love me for who I had become, for my troubles to be stilled and my 'voids' filled. Not once did I realise that what I was actually asking for, was God, . not a man of flesh and blood. It took time to realise that no man can love me like God does. No one with flesh and bones and blood and their own battle-worn souls can fill a void like God can, to heal and to make whole. But I asked him to send me one anyway!

I met my then-boyfriend six months before I qualified as a registered nurse. A gift from God, I thought, and I thanked Him for answering my prayers. My partner had grown up within the church, and so seemed to agree and understand when I told him of God's greatness in bringing him forth into my life.

How could I be so wrong when it seemed so gloriously right?

Well, therein lies a question I've been journeying to answer for some time since, finally arriving here, years later with conclusions, none of which are set in stone but all of which justify my own spiritual development and a greater understanding and appreciation for what God has been highlighting in my own life and that of many others whose path I've crossed recently.

My boyfriend and I split up two weeks after I received confirmation that I had qualified as a registered nurse. I hit my goal weight two weeks after this, mainly due to my distinct lack of appetite in having my heart torn out.

This man, I loved like I've never loved anyone before. The sun rose and set with him. I honestly saw us together forever. I believed we'd get through anything together.

It has taken me a little while to understand it, through pain, suffering and grief. But I finally have a deeper understanding, gratitude and appreciation for what happened.

God actually stepped in – this was never His plan.

During this battle, as before, I turned to my friends. To Melody. Just as she had been my rock before, she became my rock again, as she fought her own battles simultaneously, it seemed our lives had an uncanny resemblance in the patterns and synchronicities and spiritual attacks we were facing, alone yet somehow together.

Here we were in a different time and place but with that unique support and unwavering spiritual sisterhood for each other, that will move mountains. How can God not be in this?

And if God is for us, who can be against us?

In the last couple of years, things have been happening.

A new season is continuously born.

We learn, we develop, we grow, we teach, we lead.

I started to see signs and hear confirmations from people (some not even 'Christian' nor walking in faith) that I was on the right path.

That there was bigger and better coming my way.

I was in so much pain but these words somehow rang true.

I wanted my ex, but I knew deep down that we were not supposed to be together.

I started to pick apart the relationship and began to build a picture of emotional false responsibilities. Not created by this man, but by the flesh and bone and blood of every man, every woman, every personality disordered trait and every unkind spirit.

I began to understand that I saw normal whereas others saw toxicity. From trying to tell a grown man how to behave, because his actions were hurting me, I was becoming emotional because I was so very vulnerable, he was agitating and picking at my scars, and yet through all of this, I was still giving of myself with all I had.

I gave this relationship more than I had.

I gave my everything.

Every thought, every emotion, every penny in my bank, every waking smile and goodnight kiss, every touch of the hand, every stroke of the head.

I wanted this man to know how much I could give, how much I could love, but it still fell short.

I know now that it fell short because he wasn't able to receive it.

My love was too much and my emotions too deep.

My black hole impenetrable. His too.

For different reasons, but the same.

We were hurt, and both unhealed.

It took time to realise that this wasn't a unique-to-me-experience and that so many people live this way day in and day out. Unable to accept love and peace and stability.

Used to the brokenness of generational abuse and poor behaviours, we accept manipulation and gaslighting and fake personas as if it is hurtful to our spirit to accept graciousness and reality.

Twenty-first-century problems. Only foretold by God.

The realisation, the bible, the word reflects;

Only God can give all that love and stability and peace.

Only God deserves to be on that pedestal.

Only God would never throw that love back in your face.

Only God would know not to degrade you by making a mockery of your love and the gifts you give from the heart.

Only God knows how much hurt you can tolerate when you've already had your heart ripped out by the one man in your life who's supposed to love you unconditionally and without reason.

And only God will make you whole again.

No man is capable of this.

One night following this epiphany, I went to church for the first time in years.

The leader of the service came up to me as I sat waiting for Melody at the back of the room.

'You're going to be blessed tonight,' he said. And then, the service began with a bang.

Straight to the heart of me.

The message for the night... 'Turn your black holes into shining stars.'

If you don't deal with the black holes, they deal with you.

What are these black holes?

I began to cry.

Abuse is my black hole.

Physical, mental, emotional and psychological abuse.

In all its unrighteous form, in all its evil principalities, in all of its wickedness.

Abuse needs dealing with, not just in me but in the whole damn world.

There it is, without a doubt. No denial.

God was in the room and He was speaking to me.

Of all the sermons in all the world, after 18 years of being a Christian without actually ever speaking to God in a father-daughter relational capacity (with the exception of demanding He send me a man in year three of my training!), God was here to speak to me, to deal with me, directly.

I had a black hole in my soul.

A hole that I thought I could paper over.

A hole I thought I'd actually dealt with.

Not in a million years!

My void was about to be filled.

No more pain, no more suffering, just the unconditional love we're all searching for.

This black hole was responsible for all my self-doubt. For my lack of self-esteem. For my lack of belief that I would become a nurse the first time around. It saw me turn away from real godly love and turn to dead-end jobs, dead-end relationships, dead-end life. I firmly believe that the day Melody stepped into that office, God decided it was time I came home to get healed. Since that day, the hole has been gradually filling in. The event horizon of being a survivor of abuse and all that goes with it started to let love and light flow through it.

I began to lose weight. I began to believe in rock-solid foundations of friendship and love. I started to heal the hurt of past rejections. I believed in myself. I started to study, I wrote a dissertation on obesity and achieved a first in my degree. I got over surgery in super-fast time to achieve all this. I went on to fulfil His promise that I would visit Uganda, as the nurse he said I would be. I managed to open my heart to someone I believed was from God and even though I got rejected, it's okay! God is at work. I cannot deny him.

I stood at the front of the hall that night and completely broke down in the presence of my husband. He was healing me. He was holding me. He was wiping out the remains of that black hole, Sucking every atom and particle of matter out of my soul.

I could feel him breaking the bondage of abuse. I could feel him filling me with real love, giving me the gift of a father, who would love me unconditionally. He was turning me into a shining star. One that will shine brightly for his works in others. I feel it and I will live it!

A prophetic word came to me from the minister that night. A 5-fold apostle.

God told me that I hadn't missed my timing. It was just the right time. He is unburdening me of false responsibility in my life. He is taking on this care and conviction for me. He is singing a new song over my life, and in this word, God referred to me as His 'daughter'.

What a gift.

What a God.

So, today, I realise that in all of this, God has been giving me a unique insight, through His power, time and experience, all of the tools He needs me to have to do what I needed to do. And if I can hear God today, then I hear Him telling me 'you have work to do'.

This is my time, my story, and God's gift to you.

Breaking Chains that bind us with The Word. God's Word, his promise.

Addition: I picked up this chapter another couple of years on from writing it, as I once again turned to man instead of focusing on God. Having just left another toxic relationship. Also having more experiences of disingenuous family members and fake friendships and I have re-read what I wrote above and stand by it one hundred per cent. This last relationship has acted as confirmation that God has allowed me to be tested, for my iron to be forged through the fire of toxic patterns and beliefs and a lack of said faith, and with that, I have identified patterns in my own life that must end.

The conclusion here and now is, intergenerational abuse in my bloodline ends with me.

I cannot and will not allow the seeds of the devil to continue to infiltrate the seed of God within me.

I've met so many people who wear a good mask.

These relationships have kick-started my desire to spread this word afar – and to as many people as possible who are trying to understand how and why they get targeted and caught up in abusive situations with people of this ilk.

No blame, just honesty and compassion for your journey and faith as small as a mustard seed that people may read these words, see their own behaviours and toxic traits and ask for healing. Real, parental healing of the spirit. Of the inner, wounded child.

Childhood Abuse and Its Links to Mental Health

1 Samuel 22:49: "God hates abuse, viewing it as sinful and unacceptable and "delights in rescuing the oppressed."

Isaiah 41:10:10: "Fear not, for I am with you; be not dismayed, for I am your God; I will strengthen you, I will help you, I will uphold you with my righteous right hand."

The Bible speaks of mental health in various chapters. This is important to acknowledge, as we often believe that mental health is linked to the days and society in which we live. I have often linked mental health issues to such things as broken families, changing times and the increase in social networks and celebrities. However, as this passage suggests, it is actually something which God recognises as a spiritual 'presence' or 'attack' upon an individual who, it appears, has lost hope.

Psalm 42:11
"Why, my soul, are you downcast? Why so disturbed within me? Put your hope in God, for I will yet praise him, my Saviour and my God."

The mental health foundation (2017) suggests that Mental health and behavioural problems (e.g. depression and anxiety) are the primary drivers of disability worldwide, with major depression thought to be the second leading cause of disability and a major contributor to the burden of suicide and ischemic heart disease.

It is estimated that one in six people each week will experience a common mental health problem.

According to the anxiety and depression association of America (ADAA) (2016), major depression affects the way a person thinks, feels, behaves, and functions. Gorman (1996) states that approximately 85% of patients with depression also experience significant symptoms of anxiety, including panic disorder, generalised anxiety disorder, social phobia, and other anxiety disorders.

Women's Aid (2016) identify that abuse (both in childhood and in adult life) is often the main factor in the development of depression, anxiety and other mental health disorders, and may lead to sleep disturbances, self-harm, suicide and attempted suicide, eating disorders and substance misuse.

The emotional distress caused by abuse can often be exacerbated by current partners, extended family, friends or even those in leadership or mentoring positions in our lives.

Some examples of abusive behaviours include;

- Saying you're 'mad', 'crazy', 'sensitive', 'insecure' and using this as a weapon against you, your discernment and your instincts about any given situation.

- Speaking for or on behalf of you, with limited or half-truths such as 'you know you get confused/you're not very confident/you don't understand the issues'.
- Telling you you're wrong for being analytical, for delving deeper than the average person would to ensure you don't get 'hurt', 'used' or end up in the victimhood you so desperately fought to get out of once already.
- Deliberately misleading or confusing you with words, actions or morals that don't align.
- Undermining you when you disclose the abuse or ask for help: 'You can't believe her – she's mad', 'she's crazy', 'you're all the same', 'you must've done something to deserve it' etc …

These tactics almost certainly add to already deep-rooted stressors, And that is not okay, because if we give these things a voice in our lives, they become a catalyst for an ongoing cycle of mental health issues that feed into our psyche and keep us living in fear and within the shadows and confinement of anxiety, stress and further biological hardship.

This is not who we are, nor who we were ever meant to be.

Nobody in this world deserves to struggle with mental health problems. Whether the victim of abuse or not. And it is important to understand that the source of mental health often stems from the bio-psycho-social infrastructure of the world in which we participate. To cut this down into more understandable chunks that piece the jigsaw together would be beneficial.

Biologically, depression and anxiety are caused by a chemical imbalance in the brain, and this is what most drug treatments are based on. In many cases, there is a reduction in certain neurotransmitters found (serotonin and norepinephrine) which causes the symptoms of both disorders.

Serotonin and norepinephrine reuptake inhibitors (SNRIs) are a class of medications that are effective in treating depression and anxiety. SNRIs ease depression by ultimately affecting changes in brain chemistry and communication in brain nerve cell circuitry known to regulate mood, in order to help relieve depression.

Willis, J. (2007) states that serotonin brings about calmness, contentment, happiness and satisfaction, so it is in effect a mood enhancer. However, in increased amounts, it can stimulate nervous tension, heart palpitations and an inability to concentrate or perform.

Norepinephrine neurotransmitters affect the way we feel about given situations at the time we are experiencing them. If these are not available when needed, to restore emotional balance, then ill feelings can manifest.

Perkins, C. (2016) acknowledges that when a child is exposed to overwhelming and continuous stressors, such as abuse, alterations to the production and release of stress-related hormones, such as serotonin and epinephrine ensue.

When these are stimulated excessively over time, the neurotransmitter receptors become unresponsive or desensitised. Adequate levels cannot, therefore, be produced and this leads to the child victim of abuse becoming an adult with depression, anxiety, stress, cravings for carbohydrates, and a limited attention span.

Psychologically, abuse can cause many different manifestations depending upon the type of abuse inflicted. For example, physical abuse can leave cuts, bruises and broken bones. These can promote fear, nervousness, shame, avoidance and internalised anger at not being able to 'stick up for oneself' or feeling that this is somehow acceptable behaviour from someone else, inflicted upon us because it was 'deserved' in some way.

Sexual abuse can manifest as a punishment, a deserved slight for 'wearing something too revealing', a lowering of confidence, a blow to any self-esteem, a purposeful act of 'love' towards the victim, a 'secret' not to be shared, a guilt-laden act of 'favouritism' from someone in a position of control or power.

Feelings of guilt, embarrassment, shame, dread, and insecurity in later life can be destructive if these issues aren't dealt with in a healthy way, and these are also catalysts for further anxieties and stressors when we are met with situations that open up old wounds or challenge us to have to face them head-on.

Socially, anxiety and depression are still seen as something which the sufferer can 'get over' merely by 'switching off' the part of their minds that deals with these afflictions.

Mental health needs to be given the appropriate level of treatment and understanding that physical health receives. Only not with medicating the patient and altering their brain chemicals and wiring. This, in essence, is one of the most dangerous roads we can go down.

Why? Because a lot of people who suffer damage to their cognitive, behavioural, psychological and emotional well-being in early childhood or adolescent years need to be given tools for healing, not tools for covering over that which is broken.

You cannot put a band-aid over a crack and expect it not to tug, pull and break at its weakest point after some time has passed. Is it fair to victims also, to have other gifts diminished because they are changing their brain's capacity to regulate itself?

Healing comes when issues are identified, analysed, broken apart and then pieced back together. The process may take many years but it is possible to become a fully functioning and 'normal' (in the sense that other adults are normal) individual.

1 Peter 5:6–7

"Humble yourselves, therefore, under God's mighty hand, that He may lift you up in due time. Cast all your anxiety on Him because He cares for you."

I believe that a fundamental part of this process is knowing that you have a creator that can and will heal you on every level of your spiritual, physical, biological and emotional journey with anxiety and depression. It is a personal belief but one that I know is real.

How do I know? Because I've lived it, and on a personal note, I am led to share some aspects of myself that I feel will resonate with other women, and other survivors of abuse, about the influences of sexual, emotional and psychological abuse on my life.

Growing up in a disadvantaged family, with an abusive father, I often felt like I was being punished in some way.

Don't get me wrong, there were many positive relationships in my life, but above all, I felt like I was suffering, and I suppose part of me sought God in this but also blamed him for not rescuing me, or for putting me in this position in the first place.

I recall being a child that had to have an adult mentality. If I don't do this, or if I don't do that, I won't be in a position to be abused. If I hide myself away, if I don't wear that, if I don't speak out, everything will be fine.

I had a duty of not wanting to be responsible for breaking my family up at the age of ten! I didn't want to be the one who gave my brothers a broken family, to take their father away, that's not fair. But that was never my responsibility or burden to bear. I was a child.

I didn't want to cause my mother pain, I felt like I should keep my mouth shut and I lived in fear of being left alone in the house with my own dad. I'd worry about my mum seeing what was going on. I was scared, I was alone and I couldn't speak out. I carried that weight which was far greater than any child should ever have to carry.

I often heard arguments play out downstairs whilst I was in bed, between Mum and Dad. I am later told of the violence of these and how my dad tried to strangle my mum with a Hoover cord and how my teenage brother had to fight him off. I was not the only child who suffered, we all did as many others do, every day.

I heard my dad shouting and cursing and I cried into my pillow knowing I could stop it if I just spoke out – the other side of the guilt I carried! This has given me what I refer to as righteous anger as an adult and I find it almost unbearable to keep quiet these days when I see any act of abuse against another, especially against a pure, innocent child.

I sat with a social worker years later and had to tell him who I wanted to live with because Mum and Dad were fighting to win custody of us. Their toxic relationship became my bedtime story, but I never knew that any of this was abnormal, not for many many years after.

I internalised all of this fear, pain, heartache, shame and guilt. I carried it like a secret backpack, laden with a heavy load.

I am a victim, but I have to be strong. I am a child but I have to be grown.

I have to survive, I have to pretend to keep this dysfunctional family functional.

I cry some more.

How can a child feel so deeply about the feelings of everyone else? This is essentially where my intense empathy kicked in.

A child crying because the people who mean the most in the world are not who they need to be and I want them to be better.

So much better.

But there is evil in my midst.

A vile, narcissistically inclined, inhumane monster who probably resides with Satan himself living under my roof with the exceptional title 'father'.

I weep and I pray.

I recall that ten-year-old little girl taking on the world by deciding to finally put my father's 'promise' to never touch me again to the test. This promise came as a result of the family moving away, to a new home and a new location, and my mother isolated from anyone and everyone she knew.

This was the first taste of my own strength of character. I recall going downstairs to get a drink of water late at night when I knew that my dad was sleeping on the couch. I think I knew, in the back of my mind or through some kind of premonition or intuition, what was going to play out, and although I can't articulate how, I just felt a great power within me. A ten-year-old feeling like she could break the might of any man who dared to abuse, use or defile her. I was a warrior that night. This was perhaps the beginning of what I'd later refer to as discernment. One of the gifts of the real father is discernment of spirit.

1 Corinthians 2:6–16 speaks of the difference between God's wisdom and human wisdom, which is observed and thought out via human capacity whereas that of God's spirit within us, the Holy Spirit, gives access to the mind of Christ.

I remember standing in the kitchen, and this disgusting excuse of a man coming up to me and trying to lift my nightdress as I took a sip of water from a glass. A rage and courage built up inside me and at that exact moment, I decided that I was not going to be that vulnerable girl anymore. I was not playing that part.

I AM A VICTIM NO MORE.

I looked that monster square in the eyes, the same brown eyes I see when I look in the mirror, as his child, his flesh, his bones, and I spoke my powerful message right into his evil soul. You will NEVER touch me again. How dare you? Who do you think you are? I pushed his hands away and, in that moment, I felt the power of God and the force of my own spirit crush whatever demon I was being held by.

The next day, my father was taken away. I found the courage to tell my mum what was happening. And I recall apologising to my eldest brother, as I felt that I had taken away his 'daddy' and that it was my fault he'd gone, my fault my family was broken. My shame to carry.

For many years after this, I battled with my confidence. Forgetting that lioness that roared inside me. For a long time, I turned to other toxic relationships as I was drawn to 'fixing' people who were broken. Not realising I was broken too, and requiring my own form of fixing.

I ate as an emotional crux. Food became my comfort blanket. When I was sad, instead of confronting it, I used food to comfort me. And I grew larger and larger. This, too, stopped me from becoming 'attractive' to men. I guess unconsciously, I didn't want to be looked at in that way. I didn't want a man's attention on me because it scared me.

At my heaviest, in my late 20s, I was a size 22 UK. I would hide behind my weight, and my low self-esteem, to avoid any kind of relationship. I have since lost seven stone, after taking my power back and deciding to live my life with a healthier and happier mindset. I did this without medication to numb my emotions. I instead began to feel them, even more intensely than I had as a child that night in bed. I didn't run from them or hide them for fear of seeming too much of something, too nice, too kind, too intimidating, too me. I feel everything, unashamedly.

I lived for so many wasted years with the sole purpose of making life easier, or more tolerable for others. I became my mum's only friend, as years of agoraphobia and lack of confidence led to her staying in the house, hiding away unless I took her out and played my card as her pillar of strength.

And this relationship has since become a balance between wanting her to be happy and wanting my own space and life. She understands this to a point, but I still carry the burden of the old faithful internalised guilt and shame reaction, as she simultaneously fights her own black holes, at age 40 each time I leave her alone or don't 'need her' too. I became her crutch for many years – and she hated being by herself. She felt lonely and isolated, the result of her own lifetime wounds and abusive relationships. This brought about a very different form of toxicity as I'd try to please her whilst trying to grow and develop friendships that already existed, as well as to meet other people and form new relationships outside of the mother-daughter dynamic. She sees it but still, it controls our relationship as I was for many years her only real friend in this world, and she was mine, living out the broken chains that bound us both from our individual but soul-tied history.

I became involved with a church group for a number of years as a teen, where the participants and leaders used manipulation and coercion to gain control of the vulnerable youth, all in the name of their own 'spiritual' parenting. These people, I recall, blamed one of the attendees of the youth group for becoming pregnant by one of the leaders. Who I should add was a married man, and yet supported him through his distress at being 'found out'. Their toxicity and my own lukewarm faith in God, due to the nature of man, turned me away from the church and distanced me from God's grace for a long time.

I recall, around the age of 20 getting into my first serious relationship, where I learned to love, but struggled with insecurity, trust and communication. I also became a part-time mother in this relationship and looked after a child every weekend for six years. This turned my focus onto, maternal desire and nurturing. In hindsight I see my own toxic traits playing out and causing more harm than good. During counselling years later I identified my own toxic trait of care-taking and thus, the absorbing of false responsibilities for wanting to 'heal' and 'help' everyone else. Everyone but me.

At age 26, after the end of this relationship, I decided that it was time to become more self-aware. To understand the psychology of it all. To acknowledge my part in all that was happening around me and to grow and mature as a person. I decided to take action in order to develop myself and my self-worth.

I read a book at the time about parents and how their own unique attributes and projections and life experiences could reflect on their children. The title of the book, ironically, was 'they fuck you up'. I must re-read this book sometime as it was a pivotal moment in my self-discovery and yet I cannot remember a word of it.

The years following the breakdown of my first relationship saw me become an analytical, process-driven individual, who deep down just wanted to understand what made people act the way they did. What caused someone to want to abuse? What caused someone to want to control? What caused someone to be violent? What caused someone to be angry? What caused someone to cheat? What caused others to accept this? The list went on.

The answers too.

Those years saw me get involved in other toxic relationships. A married man here, an emotionally unavailable man there, emotionally immature friendships and a somewhat broken-spirited divorcee.

And through each of these relationships, I dug and dug and analysed my own patterns, my own thoughts and feelings, my deep emotions, my need to blame, my need to fix and my own emotional unavailability.

Above all, my sense of unworthiness to be loved as I should be loved.

And that leads me to where I am today. Ready to share and teach, and hopefully bring peace to those of you going through the awakening of spirit and how deeply intertwined we all are, and how this can shape and strengthen or break and chain us all to our freedom or captivity in mind, body and soul.

This process wouldn't have been possible if not for the grace of God.

I have learned that rather than blaming him, through the power of prayer, he has guided me to become a minister for his work in others' lives. To empower other women who face these trials to break the chains of abuse and toxic relationships and the demons that keep you bound in them.

I refuse to be a victim of the cards I've been dealt.

I declare that I am a woman of God. A woman of love. A woman of faith. And this is my testament.

So, mental health has been a part of my life, for most of my life. I am not in any way belittling those who feel 'better' by taking medications to 'fix' the underlying issues associated with abuse or toxic relationships in their lives. I would only ever try to support those who face these battles with the mind and pour my compassion out for each and every one of you.

This is only one person's realisation – I just hope it helps someone else to overcome the chains of bondage that are given so freely yet not talked about, as if it were a sin to suffer at the plight of our own unique journeys through this life.

The following chapters will be a breakdown of my journey, where it led me in terms of trying to 'figure everything out' and will hopefully serve as an aid for others experiencing similar patterns, thought processes and experiences to come out far healthier and faster into a reality where it's all, finally, okay!

Toxic Relationships

1 Corinthians 15:33: "Do not be misled: 'Bad company corrupts good character'."

Proverbs 13:20: "Whoever walks with the wise becomes wise, but the companion of fools will suffer harm."

Psalm 1:1: "Blessed is the man that walketh not in the counsel of the ungodly, nor standeth in the way of sinners, nor sitteth in the seat of the scornful."

1 Corinthians 5:11: "But actually, I wrote to you not to associate with any so-called brother if he is a sexually immoral person, or a greedy person, or an idolater or is verbally abusive, or habitually drunk, or a swindler – not even to eat with such a person."

Many of the articles I've read online whilst trying to 'investigate' what triggers individuals to act or behave a certain way, or show a lack of character, empathy or kindness, helped me to identify that personality disorders or traits thereof are a major contributing factor and ever-present reality in our everyday relations, and they are becoming more exacerbated by the way society has been shaped and defined in recent years.

The evidence is startling when all pieced together, in that, at a guesstimate, every 1 in 5 people you meet will probably have some form of personality disorder.

To break this down, psychology has determined that some people fall into categories of disorder, ranging from mild to severe, on a spectrum similar to that seen in Autism or Asperger's, only much less accepted. These disorders are known as things such as ADHD, Cluster A and B, narcissism, sociopathy and psychopathy and different levels of these disorders can manifest in very obvious ways, but others in more subtle, covert ways across the continuum, some individuals just having traits and some, full-blown disorders.

There are many definitions of each clustered disorder online, and a quick search of the internet will provide a lot of answers to what 'issues' each disorder brings, both to the individual suffering from them and to those who have any kind of relationship with them.

Personally, I believe I have had abusive relationships with the majority cluster B personalities on the sociopathic and narcissistic spectrum, however, I will also give space to the notion that perhaps these individuals also had their own traumas which manifested in the behaviours associated with these disorders and acknowledge that I am in no position to judge or diagnose anyone.

It would be very easy for others, outside of these given relationships, to state the obvious 'everyone brands their ex a psycho' or 'maybe the relationship just wasn't right' etc., and that's a fair enough comment. However, anyone that has been, or is currently in this type of relationship, feeling the toxicity it brings, will be acutely aware that this is not a 'normal' relationship by any means.

The sociopath and narcissistic spectrum share many traits. Some of these we'll examine more closely below. Beforehand, however, it is also important to acknowledge that we all, from time to time, show traits of narcissism that can be defined as healthy narcissism, in certain situations. The traits become unhealthy when they are used to manipulate, hurt and gain at the expense of another human being.

When you first enter any kind of relationship with those on the spectrum of these disorders, they will research you thoroughly, find out what makes you 'tick' or who you really are by any means necessary (they are known to google you!), they will check your Facebook feeds and those of your friends and family, they will ask about you, ask you to delve into your own past and to spill information to them. Get to know your hurts and black holes, your wishes, wants and desires.

Once they have identified who you are internally, what drives you, what irks or triggers you, they will then use this information to almost 'become you', by 'mirroring' yourself back to you. Please bear with me while I explain this more.

The whole process of the mirroring and, what experts and bloggers call the 'love bombing' phase of abusive relationships, is to secure you as a target. It is by 'becoming you' or 'mirroring you' back onto yourself, that they become your everything very quickly. You essentially love yourself – whilst at the very core, losing yourself in the relationship.

They know how you think, what you feel, what moves you, inspires you, scares you, makes your heart skip a beat, how many children you want, where you'd like to holiday, what movies you like, and they will use it all to showcase themselves as your 'knight in shining armour' or the 'love of your life'. Inevitably, you'll feel this way in days because they are being exactly who you are and exactly what you want. Their every action is a reaction to you, your morals and values become theirs (in observational interaction at least) and they literally become the person you want them to be. At least for the time being.

We all spend a great deal of time thinking about who we are and what we want. We ensure that we act the way we wish to be treated. We become the person we want to one day attract, and it's all real.

With a cluster B however, it is and was never real. This is a person devoid of their own sense of self. There is a void where their soul is supposed to reside. It is a black hole that is impossible for anyone, outside of the wholeness and oneness of their creator, to fill. But fill it, they try, with people and validation and 'things'.

By love bombing their target, they aim to fill this void by reflecting your love back at you, so that you continually tell them how amazing they are, how much they 'get' you, how they've saved you from all your pain etc, and they absorb all of your positive energy and light. It is only when the cracks begin to show in the next phase of their abusive continuum that things begin to unravel.

Following the love bombing is the second and third phase in a pattern known as the idealise, devalue and discard pattern, which is a trademark of cluster B personality traits.

You may not believe it without doing thorough research, but they all sing from the same hymn sheet and read the same handbook when it comes to traits and character markers. A quick internet search will have you heading down a rabbit hole that will open your eyes to what we are dealing with here. It is, I believe, Satan's finest work.

Abuse hidden behind a disorder so common and yet so readily dismissed as 'the norm' in our generation, which not only blames the victims but also enables the perpetrators. People are much quicker to judge those who identify their partners as abusive as being the perpetrator when the abuser has worn such a good false mask to the masses, only turning on their real guise when the doors are firmly closed to the outside world and they are alone, with you, the one they 'love'.

The bible tells us what to expect in the last days, and we can one thousand per cent link it to this time and this very disorder, whether we're of faith or not.

The idealisation phase we learned about above usually weakens when the individual realises that their 'prey' is wising up to their schemes. Because believe it or not, underneath this love bombing, the recipient is usually also a victim of covert forms of manipulative behaviour or emotional abuse prior to the relationship with this new toxic person, perhaps most times from childhood.

Things the narcissist or sociopath start to say and do now, become increasingly strange when compared to the love bombing behaviour. A victim will usually start to notice a sharp word here or a scathing remark there usually wrapped up with an infantile laugh and an 'I'm joking' to stop them in their tracks of taking this unnecessary behaviour to heart. At least at first.

This behaviour often escalates within three months. In my last relationship, it pretty much started from week one, but my self-esteem didn't want to believe that my charming prince was actually intentional with his abusive remarks. And we must be careful here to acknowledge abuse as abuse, the 'joking' remark may work in front of the friends who visit every other week or the brother you only see each month, but hurtful words, spoken very intentionally to knock someone else's self-esteem, are abusive.

I recall being asked in the first week of this new relationship if I actually wanted a relationship or if I just wanted to have kids because I'm 33. I guess that could've been an emotionally naive thing to say on his part, as he often liked to remind me that he didn't know how to behave in a relationship, having been married to someone who 'bought him down and cheated on him' before meeting me. I swallowed this, and with it went my own self-esteem as the criticism kept coming. I admit that question doesn't seem particularly abusive, however, this was one question that began a list of others, all hitting at the parts of me he had learned were my 'triggers', all with the intent of making me feel less than, like I didn't matter or didn't know my own mind, and all so covert that I couldn't 'quite' call it out for what it was. Insidious.

The next comment was in relation to the seven stones I shed. Which, as already stated, I put on as an emotional response to being the victim of childhood abuse, where I was told by my new flame that he 'wouldn't fancy me if I was still fat'. Straight from his own mouth. I wouldn't have even been so hurt by this had I not already fallen in love with him, love-bombed and blinded by the cognitive dissonance my mind was experiencing day in and out, even as he was at the time

2–3 stone over his own healthy weight but I never in a million years would have hurt him with such a scathing remark.

I didn't say anything to these comments, in hindsight if I had, I would have been accused of 'attacking him', which he seemed eager to point out I was doing every time I felt slighted by an abusive remark and called out that behaviour as 'not okay'.

I continually brushed under the carpet the majority of hurtful things he said, so as to not make a 'big deal' out of them, or offend him, and also through fear of hurting his feelings when his story was that he himself had been so terribly hurt before. Or so he insisted.

Looking back now, I see it was his way of controlling me. I couldn't say or do anything that would make him feel or look bad in front of other people, not as I ever had this intention anyway. Every minor thing that happened in my life, even down to my friend buying me flowers for my birthday, he used it as a reflection of himself. He asked who the flowers were from and when I told him from my friend, he said, "Oh that makes me look bad, doesn't it?" All about appearance. The flowers were in fact a bunch of lilies my friend had sent me for my birthday and had not one thing to do with him.

The criticism that comes from cluster B personalities or traits thereof actually act as a projection of their own self-hatred and acknowledgement that they are in fact insecure and broken deep within. Their own faults and failings are put onto others so that they don't have to look within and deal with the things that make them less than perfect.

The majority of these people live a life of falsehood in that they come across as confident, able and above others. They showcase this by, for example, stating that they have achieved greater, experienced more and are better than you.

When I would tell stories of real-life events that had happened to me, one particular ex would state that he had done the same, only putting a spin on it that made it better than my experience. If I had helped to save someone's life at work (as a nurse, which is commonplace) then he had performed CPR and saved a life on his own. If I had a bad day, his would be much worse. If I was busy, I would get the silent treatment for an unknown time until he finished being busy. The competition that I didn't know was happening was fierce and the jealousy pathological.

I have never been once confident enough to put myself on a pedestal and when I tell these stories or relay information about myself and how my days pan out, I never inflate, brag or overcompensate, but it was as if I would never be praised or good enough because I would always fall short with this person.

The sad part is that he was somehow aware of this as in between the put-downs and criticism, I would hear half-truths of how he didn't deserve me and would never make me happy. The truth was, he had made me happy but his abusive toxic masculinity made me so deeply sad, cut to the core and brought out triggers of my own past experiences, making me lose my confidence and feel like I wasn't seen.

The major learning curve here is, that when someone tells you they don't deserve you, believe them. It's not that he didn't deserve my love, it's just that he deserved to recognise his own first. You cannot and will not ever be able to love away someone's internal pain, or personality issues. That is a job for God and the individual alone.

There is support and acceptance that can be given – but never underestimate someone's ability to pull you and your self-esteem down in the process of trying to be someone's saviour. It'll never work.

Toxic relationships can manifest in many ways and from many sources. It is not only in close relationships but in everyday encounters that you can see them play out.

Work colleagues, close friendships and even mere acquaintances.

Often, the first sense you get that something is 'off' with a person, is a strong gut feeling. I have come to learn that trusting this is vital if you are one with an empathetic nature, as it can affect you deeply without even realising it. Back to the discernment of the Holy Spirit that is freely given to all who accept Jesus into their lives.

The first thing to remember is that, even though you want to believe everyone is the same, they are not. Not everyone has the same heart, compassion and integrity you do. You will notice, or at least begin to understand, that ego plays a huge role in the lives of toxic people. The need to act up or act out is their defence against their vulnerability that is disguised and unacknowledged. It is beyond my understanding of psychology to know if this is a conscious manifestation or if it is indeed unconscious, however, it will play out in almost every interaction with those that display cluster A, B or C personality traits.

The need to be accepted, appreciated and acknowledged may transpire as inflating their sense of self, i.e. by stating that they have done more than you (or even take praise for something you have done or achieved), by ensuring they look better than you (i.e. by being the one to pay everyone's bill at the end of a meal, even though they can't afford it), or by showing jealousy and envy when you speak of your own success.

It is often so covert that you don't see it happening and it takes a long time to acknowledge that you are being told on a small scale over and over that you are not as good as they are. I guess if you are a strong person, you may be able to live with this constant state of inferiority, but one with such deep-rooted empathy and compassion, on top of a lack of self-esteem and a history of abuse, will internalise these things day after day, year after year and suffer the consequences of it.

It is important to get to a state of self-reflection and a knowing that you are good enough, you are more than good enough and you have worked hard and developed your own personality so much so that you won't let this type of personality affect you on a fundamental level.

The Bible tells us to focus on what is true and noble, right and pure. You can only do this if you live with your own belief in goodness and rid your life of toxicity wherever possible. This doesn't mean you have to cut people out, but it does mean that you have to take accountability for your dealing with such things and set firm boundaries.

We will not grow with those looking to cut down our roots or make our flowers look bland next to theirs. We will perish. Look and pray for discernment in all things and all interactions. Your creator didn't make you to be troubled and downtrodden, but to rise up and be one with the love of his acceptance.

Philippians 4:8

"Finally, brothers and sisters, whatever is true, whatever is noble, whatever is right, whatever is pure, whatever is lovely, whatever is admirable – if anything is excellent or praiseworthy – think about such things."

Psalm 34:17 NIV

"The righteous cry out, and the LORD hears them; he delivers them from all their troubles."

The most recent relationship I came out of, which made me continue to write this book with new insight and vigour followed all of these patterns to a tee. This, as I said previously, was my confirmation that I have been put to trial to learn, accept and share with others that there is an evil seed in this world which wants to wipe out the goodness of those who live in authenticity, love and light.

This relationship started as with the prior. Expressions of love very quickly, gifts, 'soul mate' status, the usual future faking with promises of marriage, living together, holidays, children, the list goes on.

This guy, it seemed, couldn't get enough of me for being 'me'.

He stated on numerous occasions how he couldn't believe a girl like me was into a guy like him and that he felt lucky and blessed to have me.

As our relationship became more 'secure' (I use that word lightly now, but at the time it seemed that way), this guy started to become more insincere.

It started in covert ways but soon became so overt I couldn't deny that I was yet again in the thick of a toxic relationship.

One day (after I sent messages which were not delivered to this guy's phone), he came to meet me and a group of my friends for dinner and stated to me in the car on the way to meet them that he had been at another girl's house during the day.

This girl was someone I knew he had previously pursued romantically and shared a kiss with and he had previously told me how she had ruined a huge part of his year prior to getting with me as she was inviting him around to her house but also her ex-boyfriend behind his back.

I quite rightly got upset with this and explained to him that I didn't feel comfortable with him spending time with this particular girl on his own, that if he had any feelings for her whatsoever then he shouldn't be seeing her, especially behind my back and with his phone off. He became very defensive but eventually apologised and said that he could see I was right and that he couldn't see or talk to this girl again.

I said that if it was only friendship and there was nothing in it romantically, then as long as he was open and honest with me about it and didn't go behind my back, then he could remain friends with her. He agreed but stated that he didn't need to see her and that he respected me enough to cut her off. My friends even told him that his behaviour that day was wrong and he agreed and said he didn't want to hurt me, and so we continued on and, so I thought, got over this hurdle.

A couple of months into the relationship and after a trip overseas, this guy was adamant that he'd like us to move abroad. We had discussions and even started to plan how it would work with jobs, visas and the like. Because the relationship was so wonderful, or so I thought during the 'love bombing' phase, it seemed like I had met my Mr right and that finally, I could see a future with someone who 'idealised me' (I see how wrong this is now and will discuss further in the book).

Little things then started to occur which threw me off balance. They may seem like innocent happenstance to the outside reader or observer, but I know these things were set up to make me feel insecure or jealous. I can see how anyone who hasn't been in one of these toxic relationships would read that and think I sound like the crazy one (which is what these people want others to believe) but trust me, those with this covert illness really can, and do, play vicious and vindictive mind games.

One such thing that began to happen was that this guy would plant seeds of doubt in my head and then blame me for becoming suspicious or for stating that his behaviour was unacceptable, trying to burst my boundaries by chipping away at them so that his behaviour wasn't the real issue, my response to it was, a typically abusive trait. For example, he used to tell me that he had 'flirty banter' with a girl from work, but 'she's married' and there's nothing in it, it's just fun. He later admitted to having 'flirty banter' with the girl whom I mentioned above (let's not forget he told me he would never talk to her again and cut her off) for the entirety of our relationship behind my back.

When I found out he had been messaging this girl again, and asked him to see the messages (he gladly handed his phone over to me – I never 'looked' at it behind his back) he was texting her about 'doing her up the arse' and 'bringing the squirty cream round'. Upon seeing these messages I told him that this was disgusting behaviour and he actually grabbed the phone off me, turned it around on me 'you see if you've already made your mind up what's the point in looking' and blamed me for being insecure. Wow.

This guy also used to look at other girls whilst out with me. Don't get me wrong, I know guys look! But this was done to get me off balance because he wanted a reaction from me. The married woman whom he bought up every so often 'just happened' to be at a random pub he took me to one Sunday afternoon, funny how the week before he had told me he was reading emails between the staff from his IT job, so he knew full well she would be there, but pretended to me it was just a coincidence and even said 'it's just the universe's way of saying if this happens in future it's nothing to worry about'. Yeah, the guy was just full of manipulative head games.

He would come home sometimes in an obvious bad mood and when I asked what was wrong, he'd say that he felt annoyed because his friends from work had gone out and he couldn't go. When I asked what he meant he said that he knew I would 'be funny' if he went so, he decided not to go. Blaming me for something that hadn't even happened and setting the scene for the next time this would potentially occur, no doubt.

I tried to explain several times to this grown man that he didn't need to ask permission to go out, and that the only time I'd ever gotten funny with him for going out previously is when he said he was going to make dinner prior to me going on a night shift and he had turned up late with no food. He didn't want to go out but was blaming me for keeping him in. Utterly bizarre twisting of the narrative, and all done in a way to keep you off balance, second-guessing and doubting your own sense of sanity. I knew my behaviours and interactions didn't compute with what he was trying to make me believe and thus, the cognitive dissonance kicked in again, always just a little confused – enough to doubt whether this was indeed me, or him.

In the months that followed, this guy started to act aloof, cold and distant, but like I said previously it was so covert and mixed in with 'love bombing' by purchases of gifts etc. that I found the cognitive dissonance almost a normality. One minute, we'd be happily in love, the next, he would be withholding affection. It was as if I was being punished for things, I had no idea were happening, not knowing who I would be dealing with one moment to the next.

One night out of the blue, this guy blew up and stated to my face that the love had gone and he didn't want our house, the relationship or me anymore. This came exactly 24 hours after he was declaring his undying love for me and stating that he couldn't imagine his life without me.

I proceeded to pack some belongings, to leave the home we had only shared for three months and leave to spend some time away from the situation. At this point, he suggested that I shouldn't leave and he should seek therapy.

This was the first time I knew (or at least finally accepted and allowed myself to believe) of his 'mental health' issues, later self-professed.

He spent this week staying at the girl's house whom he said he wasn't in contact with during our entire courtship, but told me he was with a workmate.

Later that same week, he said that he did love me, that he wanted us to work out and that he would seek counselling.

Within the two weeks, I returned to give this relationship a chance, I discovered he had been messaging this girl the whole time, seeing her behind my back during our relationship and also downloading copious amount of porn on his PC (which, by the way, he gave me verbal permission to look at in order for me to know that I could 'trust him', never having requested this).

I left the guy and began to unpick the remnants of yet another toxic and psychologically abusive relationship. And yes... to regain my relationship with the God I had put last, for the last time.

The final part of the personality disordered or toxic abuse cycle is called the discard phase. This is where a decision is to be made, usually by the victim. See, an abuser can discard you by using techniques such as passive aggression, silent treatment or a 'trial' discard. This is where you either break the bondage of the abuse-cycle or continue in its grasp.

The more times around the cycle the more trauma bonds are created, meaning that you become less and less your authentic self, and more and more a pawn controlled by an abuser.

The abuse cycle can be found on many an internet search and will be talked about in further detail in this book, but one thing is for certain; you will not be discarded by an abuser unless YOU decide to get out or to gain strength to stand up for yourself and to get the hell out of dodgy. It is said that you always play one of 3 parts in abusive relationships, the persecutor, the rescuer or the victim. I had decided a long time ago I was no victim, but I had allowed myself to fall heavily into the rescuer archetype.

The rescuer always wants to help, to heal, to caretake. Going out of their way to make others feel special or good about themselves all whilst neglecting their own needs.

The typical co-dependent. Not quite the typical enabler as I (mostly) always felt that righteous anger flared up when something wasn't wholly moral or just, however, I played the part of rescuer well enough to stay bound by the chains of this abusive dance, and I paid a hefty price. I have learned over the years that to be fully healed is to remove oneself from any relationship that shows signs or traits of personality disordered, abusive and toxic behaviours. I appreciate it is not always easy and some people in our own lives we would struggle to fully 'cut off', and I'm by no means asking anyone to do that, but if you wish to find peace and look after yourself, you have to accept that you have a responsibility to set firm boundaries and move away from these dynamics.

It is only with God's grace, spiritual discernment and self-belief that you can identify how to live a life of peace and potentially heal and save yourself from such deep seeded pain of becoming, or remaining, entangled in this web of evil.

Personality Disorders

1 Timothy 3:2–5: **"People will be lovers of themselves, lovers of money, boastful, proud, abusive, disobedient to their parents, ungrateful, unholy, without love, unforgiving, slanderous, without self-control, brutal, not lovers of the good, treacherous, rash, conceited, lovers of pleasure rather than lovers of God – having a form of godliness but denying its power. Have nothing to do with such people."**

Delving into psychology as an amateur throws up many questions, however, it is important to note that one doesn't necessarily need a qualification to gather information about, or indeed see traits in others or themselves.

Analysing many different sources, both academic and personal blogs, has helped me to identify what motivates others to display certain characteristics and character traits.

I have already set the scene of some clustered personality traits in the previous chapter, I will now provide more information about the traits of such individuals. It is not my intention to state that those displaying such personalities do not deserve your friendship, time or love, it is merely to identify how their traits can affect you in your own growth and in the search for self-actualisation, self-esteem and self-love.

A psychological theory, proposed by Abraham Maslow in 1943, states that every human being has the need to feel respected and feel self-esteem and self-love and be accepted and valued by others. Those with low esteem and self-worth will often seek validation from others and become needy for respect and glory. This, however, will not fill the void until they fundamentally accept their true self and become aware of and regulate their own sense of self. In my opinion, by accepting that they are a creation of God, that they are accepted and were created in his image and loved, unconditionally in spite of themselves. However, a lack of self-insight and self-love and perhaps a rejection of all of the fruits of the spirit in need of constant regulation of the underlying amoral attributes of their behaviours deny God – and all that is just and morally acceptable. We could argue this is sinful, perhaps demonic in nature, or classify it as a mental health disorder. I cannot do that, but God can easily link science and religion together and by his word, he does just that.

Doctors and Psychologists use a diagnostic manual called The Diagnostic and Statistical Manual of Mental Disorders (DSM-5), to help diagnose mental health conditions. There are three main clusters of personality disorders; being;

Cluster A: Who may find it hard to relate to others or behave in a way that others consider odd, eccentric, or paranoid.

Cluster B: Who may find it hard to regulate their emotions, causing many relationship problems. They may behave in a way to be perceived as overly emotional, dramatic, or erratic.

Cluster C: Who may be seen by others as antisocial or withdrawn, with high anxiety or fearful reactions (Burgees, L. 2018).

Concentrating mainly on cluster B personality disorders highlights that there are four specific types which include; Antisocial personality disorder (ASPD), Borderline personality disorder (BPD), Histrionic personality disorder (HPD) and Narcissistic personality disorder (NPD).

The following characteristics are described by mentalhelp.net (2016) online resource as follows;

Those with antisocial personality disorders show traits such as a complete disregard for the rights, opinions and beliefs of others and can present as hostility and aggressive behaviours, deceptive actions and manipulative behaviour. These individuals often place themselves in risky situations and act on impulse. Often those with ASPD feel no remorse for their actions or will blame a victim for their own actions.

Those with histrionic personality disorder show an excessive need for attention and may come across as being surrounded by drama. This can manifest as flirtatious or seductive behaviours, often flamboyant or theatrical. Emotional expression is vague and shallow, showing insincerity to those most aware of their presence. These people are often uncomfortable being alone however their personality traits often get in the way of meaningful deep relationships.

Those with narcissistic personality disorder have a great sense of entitlement but a low sense of self-worth. They often believe they are due special treatment and have fantasies of success and power. There are differing manifestations of narcissism, with people often identifying it via a larger-than-life ego, however, it can also be very covert and difficult to spot to those merely acquainted with such an individual.

These individuals may come across as arrogant, haughty, and condescending. The realisation that these individuals do not have exceptional or above-average human ability can cause a great deal of guilt and shame, which can be taken out on others. There is a great lack of empathy, compassion and understanding for others which creates superficial relationships, devoid of real intimacy.

Those with borderline personality disorders show intense, often unstable emotions and moods. They frequently show impulsive behaviours and involve themselves in substance abuse, self-injury, risky sexual behaviours and binge eating. They can often judge themselves and others as all good or all bad, leading to an unstable sense of self and a lack of consistency.

The intense emotional reactions these people feel can lead them to experience distress which is difficult to control thus leading to impulsive self-sabotaging behaviours.

It is important to note that, from time to time, everyone can exhibit some examples of those listed, and as previously discussed a healthy degree of narcissism, in particular, is normal, however, a diagnosis of a personality disorder is dependent upon these being inflexible and should only be performed by an experienced professional.

The main focus of listing these evidenced traits is to show the reader that living with, or being surrounded by those who have these traits can be detrimental to our own mental well-being. Especially for those who have high empathetic tendencies, as the feelings and projections of others will be internalised and cause distress.

Being the survivor of abuse often leaves a person with difficulties in functioning in healthy ways in areas such as eating, sleeping, processing emotions, studying, interpersonal relationships and mental health. Understanding the effect of abuse can help the survivor process past experiences and deal with current challenges.

A child experiencing abuse often has difficulty processing normal feelings as they can feel abandoned, ignored or unloved, often by those who are the main caregiver. The child's thought pattern cannot process this information, and thus in adulthood it often transpires that the individual has inwardly directed feelings of shame, anger and guilt towards themselves. This can lead to anxiety, self-blame and helplessness.

When linked to the dynamics of those displaying personality disorders, and the cycle of abuse as mentioned in the last chapter, it is easy to see how the survivor of abuse can become a victim of a personality-disordered individual. Not necessarily through purposeful interaction on the part of the cluster B individual, but by the extent to which their personalities will affect the survivors' already diminished sense of self-love.

If we take for example the narcissists need to be superior, we will see that the survivor of abuse will feel unworthy, unloved or generally 'pulled down' by the dynamic. Thus the survivor will internalise these feelings more so than others and begin to lose much work on self-esteem in the process.

Survivors can have trust issues as a result of their perpetrators being those who were meant to protect them, and therefore can find it difficult to sustain relationships.

Projected messages such as 'you have no value' or 'you can't tell anyone' can underpin their belief systems even through adulthood and cause low self-esteem or poor self-confidence.

Rebuilding this self-esteem and confidence, therefore, needs to be a priority, so anything that wishes to counteract or diminish that needs to be addressed.

This is where as an adult, you choose what people you allow in your circle and what boundaries are healthy. The Bible also warns us of the need to avoid those who will erode your identity by saying;

Titus 3:10–11
"As for a person who stirs up division, after warning him once and then twice, have nothing more to do with him, knowing that such a person is warped and sinful; he is self-condemned."

Ephesians 4:29
"Let no corrupting talk come out of your mouths, but only such as is good for building up, as fits the occasion, that it may give grace to those who hear."

Romans 16:17
"I appeal to you, brothers, to watch out for those who cause divisions and create obstacles contrary to the doctrine that you have been taught; avoid them."

Matthew 18:15–17

"If your brother sins against you, go and tell him his fault, between you and him alone. If he listens to you, you have gained your brother. But if he does not listen, take one or two others along with you, that every charge may be established by the evidence of two or three witnesses. If he refuses to listen to them, tell it to the church. And if he refuses to listen even to the church, let him be to you as a Gentile and a tax collector."

Psychology

Strictly, theology is the study of God (from the Greek Theos) whilst psychology is the study of the mind (from the Greek psyche).

Romans 8:5–6: "For those who live according to the flesh set their minds on the things of the flesh, but those who live according to the Spirit, the things of the Spirit. For to be carnally minded is death, but to be spiritually minded is life and peace."

I am not a psychologist and have only limited educational background of such, as part of the bio-psycho-social aspect of the nursing profession and my own methodical research of this plight, however, I believe that God has given me a gift and a purpose for understanding and educating people of this complex personality disordered principality, through lived experience rather than qualification. As such, I write less from quantitative study but from qualitative experience and hindsight, attempting to fit the pieces of a rather elusive jigsaw puzzle together to make some sense of the world in which we reside. I hope that it at least lights a fire for others to delve into the depths of self-actualisation and to tie in the workings of the mind with the expansive love of the creator and indeed the universe that is alive inside and outside every cell of our being.

Psychology refers to clustered personalities as disorders characterised by unpredictable relations, interactions and thinking patterns which result in erratic patterns of behaviour that may be regarded as threatening, erratic or disturbing.

It is not my intention to stigmatise those with clustered personalities, merely to share with the reader information that I deem appropriate to share from a spiritual standpoint to protect those who need support after dealing with someone who displays these clustered traits and/or behavioural patterns, as the victim of such will often be left in a state of perplexity, possibly with PTSD or other related symptoms of abuse and a need for answers.

I have personally had to go on a very dark journey to overcome the diabolical effects of abuse, stemming from what I believe is in part spiritual warfare and seed-ship, and in this chapter, I will try to explain why I conclude this to be the case.

Over the past few years, whilst identifying certain aspects of personality disorders, I have read countless articles about what scientists say, what psychologists say, what those with the disorder say (yes there are self-professed 'narcissists' out there selling books and creating YouTube videos in our 'best interests' to teach us about their disorder) and I have come to the conclusion that these personality traits are both a spiritual AND flesh and blood issue.

When nature vs nurture comes into question, scientists and psychologists alike determine that personality disorders are long-standing, rigid patterns of thoughts and behaviours that have a link to genetics, abusive environments and long-standing patterns of abuse.

The person who we can identify as having traits of cluster B personality, displays behaviours such as the following:

Lying
Entitlement
Arrogance
Gaslighting
Control and command
Jealousy and envy
Secrecy
Triangulation
Cruelty
Dysfunctional emotional response
Low emotional empathy
Hypersensitivity to criticism
Exploitative
Mask of perfection
Manipulation
Blame Shifting
Deception
Multiple masks dependant on audience
Aggressiveness or anger
Impulsive
Reckless
Paranoid of others perception of them
Inability to be alone
Needs to be constantly busy
Wishes to create drama
Overly sexual or provocative

Delusions of grandeur
Lack of empathy
Strong need for validation

Psychologists relate these behaviour patterns to symptoms seen in the survivors of relationships with those demonstrating cluster B personality also, by stating that this can affect them in several ways – these include:

Self-blame Echoism
Insecure attachment styles
Fierce independence
Extreme narcissism
PTSD

So we can see here that, in terms of flesh and blood, a narcissistic parent for example could create a narcissistic child OR a child with severe PTSD and insecure attachment styles (as in, a child who suffers for their father's sins no matter which way they are nurtured).

I personally believe that my abusive father was on the cluster B spectrum. Can I prove this? No. But I can see those traits and relate them to such.

I can also acknowledge and wholeheartedly believe that this has led me to become one that has self-blamed, echoed (being overly sensitive and empathetic means I put others' needs ahead of my own for the majority of my life), become insecurely attached (having anxiety at putting myself in someone else's hands) thus leading me to a fierce sense of independence and developing that righteous anger that I previously discussed.

I also show traits of PTSD from exposure to those with undeniable personality disorder traits, which manifest as hypervigilance, hyperawareness, anxiety and fight or flight reactions.

Are my developed traits any different to those who develop clustered disorders? In some respects no, we are all a product of our childhood and traumas, however, my reactive traits are for self-preservation, not self-importance or self-gain and I can identify with others and show compassion, support and love. Those fruits of the spirit that God grants us when we go to him with acceptance of what he can do to change and heal and save us, from ourselves and those who trigger the black holes within us.

In viewing this in line with spirituality we can see that God has forewarned us about the types of people that possess these traits, in order to protect us from harm. If we can link narcissism for example as a hereditary trait, then God can show us how to deal with that seed and throw it out. After all, we all have a choice.

Psychology also gives us a further visual representation of the abuse cycle; this goes as follows:

1. Tension building: walking on eggshells, tension builds and there is a feeling of broken communication, where the abusive partner (spouse, child, parent, friend) will talk in 'word salad' whereby no conclusions to any questions are resolved nor positive outcomes identified. The victim will often feel they need to placate the perpetrator so as to bring calm or resolve to a situation. The victim in this

phase feels their voice isn't heard or their opinions unimportant and a decrease in self-esteem ensues.

2. Incident: An incident of abuse occurs, whether verbal, physical, psychological, emotional or physical. There is anger in this stage, as well as blame shifting, where the abuser will suggest that you are at fault for something they've done or are doing, or will project issues onto you that don't resonate with what you know to be your personality traits. There can also be threats or intimidation. This leads to diminished confidence and a need for a normally functioning individual to try to make the abuser understand that they are not what they are being accused of, rather than identifying that the abuser is, in fact, trying to get you to own the issues they have.

3. Reconciliation: The perpetrator gives apologies, excuses, blames the victim or denies the abuse took place or says it wasn't as bad as the victim is making it out to be. A complete denial of abuse in their mind means that they are not actually guilty and therefore cannot be held accountable for their behaviour. If it wasn't done 'on purpose' (which it always is – don't fall for that) then why are we (the victims) being so 'mean' by blaming them or holding them accountable? This is where cognitive dissonance steps in.

4. Calm period: this is where the abuser is forgiven and, in an attempt, to encourage further 'supply' from the victim, they go back to the loving, caring and supportive spouse (or another close person) that they were in the beginning. They will often use this period

to shower you with loving gestures, gifts and words of comfort and apology, insisting that this is the 'real' person and the abuse that just occurred was a one-off and misunderstanding.

You can see from this list how it links in with the clustered modus operandi of 'idealise, devalue and discard'. It is not by coincidence that the two match up.

Psychology suggests that there is a disorder that makes people display these traits and like I've already suggested to a point I agree, however when you've dealt one on one with people with these 'disorders' you can see quite clearly that they actually enjoy, or get a high from behaving in this callous way.

That is not a disorder alone, that is a spiritual entity of hate and pure evil working through the flesh and blood. A lack of the fruit delivered only by God's Holy Spirit.

The Bible says in **2 Timothy 3:2** that in the end times, people will be lovers of themselves, lovers of money, boastful, proud, abusive'.

From personal experience, two particular people from my past have actually looked me in the eye and smirked as they've self-professed that they are (sorry for the language but in their own words) 'a cunt', whilst boasting about how mean they've been or how they've got away with disrespectful behaviours.

That is not a personality disorder alone, that is a spiritual principality, as The Bible tells us that "we do not wrestle against flesh and blood but against the rulers, against the authorities, against the cosmic powers of this present darkness, against the spiritual forces of evil in the heavenly places" **(Ephesians 6:10–12).**

Abusers see nothing but themselves, they are often proud, haughty, boastful and selfish.

They have no idea that there is a God who can help them because they have no idea, they have a problem. When you feel superior to others and don't feel that you have a problem, you will not seek help. This is why it is so very important for survivors of abuse to recognise that they are the only ones who can stop the cycle. The only ones aside from God.

An abusive person will not cut you off (or even if they do, they will do so to gain power and return at a later date) because they don't see that they are the issue.

They feel attacked if you point out their unnatural behaviours and will blame you for every issue that arises. You are the one who has to step away. The difficulty in doing this lies within the abuser's cycle, with the development of cognitive dissonance and trauma bonds.

Cognitive dissonance is the state in which inconsistent beliefs or attitudes, thoughts or beliefs are shaped and decisions made. When someone flips between 'Mr perfect' and 'Mr who the hell is he', it creates uncertainty. I'll discuss this more later in the book.

On one hand, you believe the love of your life is for you, he after all treats you like a queen in front of his friends, buys you nice gifts and flaunts you on his social media. But when he then pokes fun at your weight or tells you not to wear the beautiful dress you've bought because you look like a tart, or criticises the way you speak, your mind begins to falter, especially when you call out the unnecessary behaviour and then get told you're too sensitive or he was just joking.

These constant opposite behaviours create that sense of 'walking on eggshells' where you feel you cannot be who you are for fear of being either built up or torn down. This then creates a diminishing of your self-esteem, without you even realising it's happening, and you become a shell of the person you once were.

Trauma bonds are similar in that each time an abuser repeats their cycle, and you go back to the idealisation phase, you essentially become reliant on the 'idealisation' phase as you then get to 'feel' the kind of love you felt in the beginning when the mask was firmly in place and the perpetrator was actually mirroring all that is good in you, back to you.

We begin to crave this level of deep intimacy and what we see as 'love' and connectedness, negating the fact that we should never have been devalued and discarded in the first place, as a healthy relationship doesn't work this way.

They say that the average person takes seven attempts to flee an abusive relationship. I believe that this gives us enough evidence of the fact that, in the majority of cases, these people do not change. Please hear me, I'm not stating that they can't change, but that they need intervention more than counselling and therapy to do so.

They need God.

Analysing

2 Corinthians 13:5: "Examine yourselves to see whether you are in the faith; test yourselves. Do you not realise that Christ Jesus is in you – unless, of course, you fail the test?"

Romans 12:2: "Do not conform to the pattern of this world, but be transformed by the renewing of your mind. Then you will be able to test and approve what God's will is – his good, pleasing and perfect will."

Lamentations 3:40: "Let us examine our ways and test them, and let us return to the Lord."

Psalm 119:59–60: "I have considered my ways and have turned my steps to your statutes. I will hasten and not delay to obey your commands."

A person with a clustered personality traits will often use remarks such as 'you over-analyse everything', 'stop overthinking', 'you're too sensitive' etc. This is a fundamental part of the abuse cycle whereby you end up questioning and diminishing your own self-esteem, as you will begin to wonder if indeed the issue is with your reaction to, rather than their actual abusive behaviour.

I recall when an ex of mine would say something cruel and when I reacted, by asking why he felt that way or became defensive to protect my psych from this insidious abuse, he would immediately shift to stating that 'I'm just joking', 'you're so emotional' etc. The blame always landed at my feet. He even expanded on this during one discussion to state that he 'doesn't do feelings' and that he was more the 'logical' one. Had I known then that he meant he didn't actually have feelings, I'd have saved myself a lot of heartache. It turns out though, that this is exactly what those with these disorders or traits don't want you to know.

Only on reflection and indeed, deeply analysing the situation following discard, can I see how this behaviour slowly but surely wreaks havoc on a person's true identity.

When you doubt your own instincts and ears, listening to the person who self-promotes as 'a nice guy' actively being mean and vindictive to others in his own words, from his own mouth, you develop cognitive dissonance.

Cognitive dissonance is the state of inconsistent thoughts, beliefs or attitudes relating to behavioural attitudes and decisions. It is this exact process which leaves you in a state of confusion when leaving or being discarded after an abusive situation, as, on one hand, you know this person (at the beginning whilst idealising and mirroring you) was presenting themselves as an honest, empathetic, caring, loyal individual, but their actions were showing you that they were in fact manipulative, jealous, controlling, vindictive and spiteful.

When the mind tries to process the abuse, it cannot merely switch either of these realities off, therefore, it keeps replaying situations like a projector rolling over and over again trying to make sense of the nonsense. This I believe is the root that leads to the anxiety and complex PTSD symptoms identified in many, many survivors of narcissistic or other forms of abuse.

Only when a person comes to the conclusion that they were used, or conned by this individual, can they truly begin to heal and let go, as they realise that none of what happened was how they wished. An abuser hasn't got the same heart as you and until you realise, they are wired with a distinct lack of empathy and compassion, you cannot forge ahead and begin to heal yourself.

Let me tell you, there is nothing wrong with being analytical. Abusers make you believe there is because they don't want you to catch on to their games through logic and understanding. My most recent ex said in the heat of a discussion where he was being uncovered that I had 'so much self-worth and my intuition frustrated him'. I believe that says it all.

What person who wasn't trying to manipulate or deceive someone else would ever find someone else's self-worth an issue? Only one who has none of their own, who must beat you down in order to bring themselves up. A relationship like this is literally a soul rape and can damage a person beyond repair.

Trauma bonds are created as a result of the constant push and pull dynamics of these relationships and are formed due to intense emotional experiences with those who provoke or elicit positive or negative emotional responses through psychological or physical abuse.

Similar to Stockholm syndrome, the victim usually wants to seek comfort from the very person who has caused the trauma. It makes the victim want to return to the abuse as this is what becomes the norm due to the cycle mentioned above. As already suggested, many domestic violence articles state that it takes up to seven individual occurrences of abuse for a victim to leave their perpetrator. This is why victims also often face shame from outsiders whom they may have confided in.

People who've never been in this situation can be quick to judge and state things such as 'why didn't you just leave' or 'if it was that bad why did you go back'.

Although not done in spite, this doesn't help the survivor and adds to their guilt at their own need for vindication and also their own frustration at not being able to get away.

I believe that emotional resilience and personality disorders, and the traits of such, are something which need to be discussed from a young age, in an ever-present society which is becoming more narcissistic, to ensure the emotional needs of children, young adults and older adults alike are managed and able to overcome this destructive spirit.

Victimhood

John 5:6: "When Jesus saw him lying there, and knew that he already had been in that condition a long time, He said to him, 'Do you want to be made well?'"

Matthew 16:24: "Whoever wants to be my disciple must deny themselves and take up their cross and follow me."

I've chosen to write a chapter on victimhood for two reasons. The first one being that victimhood can be considered a trait of a covert narcissist or abusive personality-disordered individual. The second is an attempt to shine a light on the survivor and allow them to realise that they don't have to live in a state of victimhood regardless of what life has dealt them.

Let me expand on both ideas below.

When considering a toxic individual who is abusive and suffers from one of the clustered personalities (or has traits of such), it is often apparent that they enjoy or live within what are commonly referred to as 'pity plays'. These often play out as a 'woe is me' kind of relationship with other people.

Some examples of this could be when someone states that they act a certain way (which is non-negotiably abusive to a non-toxic individual) because 'they've been hurt before', thereby lining themselves up with the assumption that it's now okay for them to act shady or inappropriate as justifiable due to their own pain. Not okay.

Please allow me to be the first to remind you here that, as a survivor of abuse, you wouldn't act this way and would also question the behaviour of anyone other than the abusive party.

One way you can always calculate this in your brain whilst overcoming the victimhood associations with abuse, is to simply ask yourself the question 'is that something I would've said or done' – if your answer is no, then why are you accepting it from someone else?

If that is the case, then someone stating that they've been hurt and therefore it's acceptable for them to hurt you or others would mean that it's now okay for you to hurt them back. You see how this cycle continues? Abuse and hurt and pain and is never okay, not ever, nada.

The thing is, an abusive person wouldn't accept the kind of behaviour they dish out and would accuse you of being abusive. This happened to me when I called out an ex on his cheating, whilst he was angrily trying to get me to allow him to remain friends with the girl he'd been actively pursuing behind my back.

I asked him outright if the shoe was on the other foot, and he had read text messages to another man and I had been trying to coax him into a liaison with me. Would he now be okay with me trying to remain friends with him whilst staying in a relationship with you (the perpetrator). Of course, he said no, but couldn't quite connect the meaning of what I was saying, instead labelling me 'vindictive' because I wouldn't allow his abuse to continue once brought to light. Apparently, my noticing his behaviour was worse than the act of infidelity was.

A victim mentality is one whereby the perpetrator says 'they don't know how to act in a relationship', thereby giving them enough leeway to act how they please at your expense. This was a line of another abusive partner of mine, who had not only had numerous 'relationships' prior to ours but had in fact been married for a good number of years prior to our courtship.

People exhibiting the victim mentality will blame whomever they can for their own bad behaviour.

I've had abusive and toxic people in my past blame their parents, their peer group and even myself for the vicious acts they say or do to others. This is where we need to relate back to the abuse cycle and realise that these people do not only use their techniques on their significant other but on anyone who gets in the way of what they want.

This is also the reason that we each, individually, have to explore the nuances of other people's relationships and not take what we're told by an individual to heart but to test the spirits and discern what's right and pure and truthful and just.

So many victims are the ones who keep quiet, who are smeared by the actual abuser and targeted and blamed not only by them but by their own friends and family because of this.

In regards to the survivor, for a short time after abuse, you will see these people almost 'taking on' the personality of the abuser.

This is a time when others may believe the perpetrator due to the symptoms of abuse playing out in your psyche. It has been termed 'reactive abuse' or 'narc fleas' in many articles and psychology blogs.

You may show fits of anger (when this is not who you usually are), shout, scream and become enraged by the injustice of what you've been through (or are currently escaping from).

This is a time when the abuser knows they can 'set you up' to appear as the one who is unstable. This is where many victims get labelled as 'the crazy ex' whilst they are in a grieving period of betrayal, hurt and loss.

Don't put it past a manipulator to use your reactions as a justification for them smearing your name.

Imagine you've found out information about the abusive individual that she or he may have staged so that when you call to confront them, they happen to be sitting with friends or a family member who hears your raised voice and then agrees with the perpetrator that you sound unhinged or abusive.

Please don't take that lightly as this is the kind of reaction they want. This is also why many articles you will read suggest that the best way to deal with one of these clustered personalities, once identified, is to cut off all contact, cold turkey and run for the hills (you'll hear a lot how you should never look back and believe me, in some instances, it's true).

As Maya Angelou stated in one of her famous quotes; If someone shows you who they are, believe them the first time... Here I'll add 'and get out' or at the very least set firm boundaries and test the spirit.

Also, please don't feed into the victim status or listen to uneducated people who will quote such things to you as 'hurt people, hurt people'. Yes, in theory, I guess that's true, but as I said, you've been a victim of abuse, and are you hurting anyone or just yourself? Don't lower yourself to their standards, and begin to rise out of the hell they're dragging you into.

Romans 12:2

"Do not be conformed to this world, but be transformed by the renewal of your mind, that by testing you may discern what is the will of God, what is good and acceptable and perfect."

Romans 12:18

"If possible, so far as it depends on you, live peaceably with all."

Romans 12:17–21

"Repay no one evil for evil, but give thought to do what is honourable in the sight of all. If possible, so far as it depends on you, live peaceably with all. Beloved, never avenge yourselves, but leave it to the wrath of God, for it is written, 'Vengeance is mine, I will repay, says the Lord.' On the contrary, 'if your enemy is hungry, feed him; if he is thirsty, give him something to drink; for by doing so you will heap burning coals on his head.' Do not be overcome by evil, but overcome evil with good."

Self-Hate – Self Love
(The In-between)

Genesis 1:27: "So God created mankind in his own image, in the image of God he created them; male and female he created them."

Ephesians 2:10: "For we are God's masterpiece, created in Christ Jesus to do good works, which God prepared in advance for us to do."

Ephesians 5:8: "For you were once darkness, but now you are light in the Lord. Live as children of light."

2 Timothy 1:7: "For the Spirit God gave us does not make us timid, but gives us power, love and self-discipline."

1 Corinthians 13:4–7: "Love is patient, love is kind. It does not envy, it does not boast, it is not proud. It does not dishonour others, it is not self-seeking, it is not easily angered, it keeps no record of wrongs. Love does not delight in evil but rejoices with the truth. It always protects, always trusts, always hopes, always perseveres."

Let's determine where you are right now, or where you've recently been.

What has led you to purchase this book (and probably countless others about God, faith, self-love and self-acceptance following abuse) I'm going to take a punt and state that you no longer know who you are. You've lost your sparkle. You no longer look in the mirror and smile. You feel hollow, empty and unable to get back the girl you used to be, before all this.

You blame yourself for being too nice, for giving too much of yourself away, again, to someone who used, abused and discarded you. You feel not good enough. You ask yourself what you've done to deserve this, but come up with nothing.

That my beautiful unique soul is because you did nothing wrong – and because you were everything right.

Abusive people don't choose other abusive people to have relationships with. There would be no ability to control another with the same disorder, the same temperament and the same abusive behaviours.

They choose people with unlimited compassion, empathy and a need to fix. An abuser will look for the most vulnerable person they can find. Often the issue is that through their love bombing and idealisation phase, they are filling your own vulnerability (let's take for example that you were already the victim of abuse) with unconditional love, understanding, compassion and fake empathy (all the things you need to feel 'safe') and then in the devaluation phase, tearing all of this back away from you (tearing open new scars along with old traumas in an attempt to break you).

Going back to the traits you as a victim will no doubt possess in abundance, we can look at what the bible states are these 'fruits' are, in **Galatians 5: 22–23:** "The fruit of the Spirit is love, joy, peace, forbearance, kindness, goodness, faithfulness, gentleness and self-control. Against such things, there is no law."

There is however a deceiver. The devil is a liar. Jesus speaks of this in **John 8: 37–59:** "You are of your father, the devil, and the desires of your father you want to do. He was a murderer from the beginning and does not stand in the truth, because there is no truth in him. When he speaks a lie, he speaks from his own resources, for he is a liar and the father of it. But because I tell the truth, you do not believe Me. Which of you convicts Me of sin? And if I tell the truth, why do you not believe Me? He who is of God hears God's words; therefore, you do not hear, because you are not of God."

Abusers don't hear what is true, what is righteous and just, because it doesn't serve them or their ego. It serves the one almighty God whom their spirit is in opposition with.

They live largely for self-atonement, seeking pleasure from pain, whilst lying and boastful of their deceit. This is where survivors must realise that in blaming themselves, they are in essence, claiming account for another's traits or fruits, or ability to take their own responsibility. This is unjust. We wouldn't take responsibility for someone else's success or compassion or empathy, so why would we take responsibility for their hurtful, demeaning and unacceptable behaviours, as if we are at fault?

I received a word from God from a well-renowned prophet just after the breakdown of one of these abusive relationships, about being set free from false responsibility and I fully acknowledge that God was speaking of the bondage of abuse.

I know that God can work miracles. I know that he can forgive, cleanse and make all things new, that is why I rebuke every attack from the devil telling me that I am a victim or to blame for someone else's sin.

I choose self-love because in the blood of Jesus I am set free. Every act of love sets me free. I am not in bondage like my oppressor. I am free indeed because I know God and I know love. There is no greater blessing and as the words of **Matthew 22: 25–40** state, the greatest commandments of the law are these: "Thou shalt love the Lord thy God with all thy heart, and with all thy soul, and with all thy mind. And the second is like, unto it, Thou shalt love thy neighbour as thyself." On these two commandments hang all the law and the prophets.

All the law states that love is the only way. So we cannot blame ourselves for somebody else acting out. We cannot repay hatred for hatred. We cannot live in self-victimisation, because it is against the will of our creator. Therefore, abuse is a sin.

It is up to the abuser to identify these traits within him or herself and to do the self-reflection or analysis (which let's not forget they paint as a fault in you) to overcome their disorder and find their root in God, in love.

Deuteronomy 31:8

"The Lord himself goes before you and will be with you; he will never leave you nor forsake you. Do not be afraid; do not be discouraged."

Who Are You?

Galatians 2:20: "I have been crucified with Christ and I no longer live, but Christ lives in me. The life I now live in the body, I live by faith in the Son of God, who loved me and gave himself for me."

Romans 8:38–39: "For I am convinced that neither death nor life, neither angels nor demons, neither the present nor the future, nor any powers, neither height nor depth, nor anything else in all creation, will be able to separate us from the love of God that is in Christ Jesus our Lord."

Song of Solomon 4:7 "You are altogether beautiful, my darling; there is no flaw in you."

In this chapter, we are going to identify who you are. Not only in the flesh but in the spirit.

So I'll take this forward personally and you can use this as a guide to do the same.

You'll see how I relate this to my backstory.

How my life and works have evolved over time in line with God's plan for my life. How the devil has lied to me and how God's grace has covered me time and time again.

How love will defeat evil and how a mindset can shift from self-blame to self-love by breaking down the lies against your life from the father of sin.

I hope that by doing this, the opportunity for you to reflect and determine what great attributes you have in your own life can be determined and related to the false accusations placed upon you by the abuser and from the father of lies.

Who am I?

In the flesh:

I'm longed for a daughter, for a mother who loves me and a father who was an abuser. Possibly one with narcissistic personality disorder who regardless of a diagnosis, used covert manipulation, lies and deceit, physical, emotional and sexual abuse to control and pervert his own flesh and blood.

In the spirit:

"I am a child of God." **2 Corinthians 6:18**

"Because I have faith in Jesus." **Galtaians 3:26**

"I am a gift from the womb and a reward." **Psalm 127:3**

"No one who is born of God practices sin, because His seed abides in him; and he cannot sin, because he is born of God. By this, the children of God and the children of the devil are obvious: anyone who does not practice righteousness is not of God, nor the one who does not love his brother." **1 John 3:9–10**

God is showing me here that I am his daughter because I chose to believe that I was a gift and reward, created in his image and with faith in Jesus. I, therefore, choose righteousness over sin because I do not belong to the father who abuses. I belong to the father who gifted me breath in my lungs, love in my heart and the choice to do good over evil.

In the flesh:

I am a woman who has been put through tests and trials. I have fought battles against flesh and blood with the mindset of a broken child until I discovered who I am in the spirit. I have lived for too many years always scared to speak out against those who have tried to dominate or rule over me with vicious words or actions or lies.

In the spirit:

*"In the world, you will have tribulation. But take heart; I have overcome the world." **John 16:33***

*"And after you have suffered a little while, the God of all grace, who has called you to his eternal glory in Christ, will himself restore, confirm, strengthen, and establish you." **1 Peter 5:10***

*"She opens her mouth with wisdom, and the teaching of kindness is on her tongue." **Proverbs 31:26***

*"She is more precious than jewels, and nothing you desire can compare with her. Long life is in her right hand; in her left hand are riches and honour. Her ways are ways of pleasantness, and all her paths are peaceful. She is a tree of life to those who lay hold of her; those who hold her fast are called blessed." **Proverbs 3:15–18***

In the flesh:

I am a nurse. I was called via prophecy to this career. I have since received confirmation from God via prophecy that

I am not only a nurse but that he has greater promises for me, yet to be established.

I believe God wants me to release this book in line with the calling on my life. A recent teaching I was listening to on YouTube by a well-known minister spoke of two nurses in a hospital looking after his mum, and the difference in their care (or calling) was that the one who had been through the same experience with her mother was able to give a different level of care to the patient than the one who hadn't. This leads me to believe that God wants me to release this word as a stepping stone to the beginning of ministry for survivors of abuse, to step up and claim your victory.

In the spirit:

"For I know the thoughts I think toward you, says the Lord, thoughts of peace and not of evil, to give you a future and a hope." **Jeremiah 29:11.**

"And we know that all things work together for good to those who love God, to those who are called according to His purpose. For whom He foreknew, He also predestined to be conformed to the image of His Son, that He might be the firstborn among many brethren The 'brothers' and 'sisters' are those who are a part of the church of Christ." **Matthew 23:8; Matthew 12:50; Hebrews 2:10–18; Romans 8:28–29.**

"Before I formed you in the womb I knew you, and before you were born, I consecrated you; I appointed you a prophet to the nations." **Jeremiah 1:5**

In the flesh:

I am an overcomer, I have won battles against that which was sent to destroy and diminish me. I use my hurt to heal, my pain to prosper and my brokenness to fix. I have suffered through depression, anxiety and PTSD as after-effects of abuse but I know that God is greater than the woes of my flesh and mind.

In the spirit:

"The LORD is my light and my salvation – whom shall I fear? The LORD is the stronghold of my life – of whom shall I be afraid?" **Psalm 27:1**

"Cast all your anxiety on Him because He cares for you." **1 Peter 5:7**

"Blessed is the one who perseveres under trial because, having stood the test, that person will receive the crown of life that the Lord has promised to those who love him." **James 1:12**

"My grace is sufficient for you, for my power is made perfect in weakness." **2 Corinthians 12:9**

"You, dear children, are from God and have overcome them because the one who is in you is greater than the one who is in the world." **1 John 4:4**

In the flesh:

I have been broken-spirited, broken-hearted. I have been so in the thick of cognitive dissonance that I didn't know which way was up. But I have also learned that fleshly desires will never fill that void inside. Only God can do that. Therefore I have also proclaimed I was a sinner, I put man before God and I have asked for forgiveness as we all should. I am not perfect, I never claimed to be. In my sin, I suffered, just as abusers suffer in theirs. We all have to accept the one true love to overcome our weaknesses and be made perfect in God's forgiveness.

In the spirit:

"He heals the broken-hearted and binds up their wounds." **Psalm 147:3**

"Blessed are the poor in spirit, for theirs is the kingdom of heaven. Blessed are those who mourn, for they shall be comforted. Blessed are the meek, for they shall inherit the earth. Blessed are those who hunger and thirst for righteousness, for they shall be satisfied." **Matthew 5:2–12**

1 John 1:9

"If we confess our sins, he is faithful and just to forgive us our sins and to cleanse us from all unrighteousness."

Losing What No Longer Serves You

Philippians 3:12–14: "Not that I have already obtained this or am already perfect, but I press on to make it my own because Christ Jesus has made me his own. Brothers, I do not consider that I have made it my own. But one thing I do: forgetting what lies behind and straining forward to what lies ahead, I press on toward the goal for the prize of the upward call of God in Christ Jesus."

Romans 8:28: "And we know that for those who love God all things work together for good, for those who are called according to his purpose."

Abuse, in all its forms, makes us feel as though we are bound up in chains, a lot of survivors have an overwhelming guilt surrounding them which stops them from claiming the power which is rightfully theirs. Guilt can make a survivor more susceptible to remaining stuck in patterns and cycles, always trying to please and fix others, rather than doing the work on self that is required to break free of bondage and grow in God's works and purpose.

God can and will break chains. You just need to fully accept that you are healed. Cut off that which no longer serves you. Go completely no contact with anyone who shows signs of abusive behaviour, where you can, or limit your dealings with those you cannot fully break loose from and don't react emotionally to them in any way shape or form. Set firm but righteous boundaries.

People who abuse enjoy or take pleasure from pain, reaction and emotion from your spirit as previously discussed. If you ask God to step in and seek him first, He will support you, lift you up and change your destiny.

You have to find your inner child, the one whom God knew even before you were of flesh and blood, and you have to protect and guide it as you would a real child. Place your inner child into God's hands and let Him guide you both to a place of peace, joy, hope and freedom.

The secret is this, you have to find your purpose, even in the midst of your pain. God didn't create us to be downcast, nor to live a life of pain due to others' sinful ways.

God created each and every one of us with a purpose and a destiny. Will you allow that to be diminished by the devil? Or will you find that little light within you that just needs some belief, some nourishment and some faith to be released?

Those that choose hate will perish. They may think there is no ramification for their evil wicked way, but the Lord reminds us that He sees their works and that He will avenge them.

Romans 2:8–12 tells us that 'for those who are self-seeking and who reject the truth and follow evil, there will be wrath and anger, There will be trouble and distress for every human being who does evil: first for the Jew, then for the

Gentile; but glory, honour and peace for everyone who does good: first for the Jew, then for the Gentile'.

For God does not show favouritism. All who sin apart from the law will also perish apart from the law, and all who sin under the law will be judged by the law'.

God is the only one who can judge. But He gives us the power to discern and to take heed of His warning about those of wickedness and guides us by his Word and the Holy Spirit.

1 John 4:1

"Beloved, do not believe every spirit but test the spirits to see whether they are from God, for many false prophets have gone out into the world."

1 Corinthians 13:1–13

"If I speak in the tongues of men and of angels but have no love, I am a noisy gong or a clanging cymbal. And if I have prophetic powers, and understand all mysteries and all knowledge, and if I have all faith, so as to remove mountains, but have no love, I am nothing. If I give away all I have, and if I deliver up my body to be burned, but have no love, I gain nothing. Love is patient and kind; love does not envy or boast; it is not arrogant or rude. It does not insist on its own way; it is not irritable or resentful."

Matthew 10:16

"Behold, I am sending you out as sheep in the midst of wolves, so be wise as serpents and innocent as doves."

Many people will enter your life dressed as a wolf in sheep's clothing.

Pertaining to be meek and mild and yet with an air of deceptiveness, waiting to bite the hand that feeds them. This is often referred to as the 'Jekyll and Hyde' personality, or duality and another trait of those with clustered personality traits and disorders.

Many articles refer to this as a person's mask, each one chosen and worn depending on which audience they are in the presence of.

It is quite clear after spending considerable time with a person displaying abusive or narcissistic tendencies that this is happening.

Although, at first, it may appear someone does this because they have low self-esteem or are trying to appease people, with the disordered individual, it is another way by which they mirror their targets.

For example, one previous partner of mine used to be extravagant in front of his friends, paying for expensive meals for every member of a group or for everyone's drinks at a party, even though he was in a huge amount of debt (I didn't know about the debt until we had split up), however when I spoke to him about this he stated that I was 'attacking him', rather than seeing that I was merely concerned about him.

As it transpires, his mask of superiority was taking on the debt from the meal in a bid to appear grandiose and like the 'nice guy' he wanted everyone to believe he was.

The same guy uttered contempt towards me for buying him an inexpensive whisky whilst on a night out with his business partner and her new beau, and then later when he received a glass from said beau, looked at me and stated quite loudly 'see, this is real whisky'. I assume to put me in my place and show his superior taste and attitude. What makes me laugh a little harder about this particular incident now is that at the time I was a student struggling to live on a bursary of £340 per month, but I was expected to live up to 'Mr egos' £10 a glass whiskey expectation or be made to feel 'less than' because I couldn't. Thankfully, I didn't need to get myself into debt to prove myself to anyone and continued to buy the 'lower-end range' whiskey!

These types of behaviours are haughty and proud and offend my spirit as I wouldn't act like that towards another. It may seem innocent enough in itself, but when it is constantly belittling put-downs, it affects you in a mighty way.

You feel as though you're the abusive one when all you're doing is loving, giving and trying to support, help and appease someone who will never be grateful or satisfied.

This is why we must let go of people who act in this manner, as a protection for our very sense of self. As perseverance. As a stand for what's right and noble and just, or set firm and righteous boundaries whilst keeping them in your prayers.

Hebrews 6:10 reminds us that God is not unjust; he will not forget your work and the love you have shown him as you have helped his people and continue to help them.

It's a Choice

Psalm 11:5: "The Lord tests the righteous, but his soul hates the wicked and the one who loves violence."

Colossians 3:8: "But now you must put them all away: anger, wrath, malice, slander, and obscene talk from your mouth."

Luke 6:45: "The good person out of the good treasure of his heart produces good, and the evil person out of his evil treasure produces evil, for out of the abundance of the heart his mouth speaks."

Proverbs 22:24: "Make no friendship with a man given to anger, nor go with a wrathful man."

Romans 12:21: "Do not be overcome by evil, but overcome evil with good."

This chapter I wish to write for those who identify with having one of the personality disorders (or traits of such) identified in this book.

I have not written this book to attack anyone suffering from clustered disorders or traits thereof. I have merely identified the hallmarks of the disorders and how they scientifically and psychologically mirror and reflect the cycles of abuse and can be identified as a distinguishing factor of those who chose this to be their all-encompassing way of life.

I call it a choice because I thoroughly believe some traits of it are.

Yes, it can be a disorder, on a continuum, but many still have the ability to identify right behaviours from wrong behaviours, even if their neural pathways have not yet developed the mechanisms needed to react appropriately in the moment. People have a choice whether to be defined by this disorder or whether to be a better person.

In order to do better, we need to identify that we were created by an omnipotent, omnipresent God. We are not all-powerful and our works will be seen and judged just as everyone else's. If an individual sincerely gets pleasure from the pain of others they need deliverance.

I don't wish to be harsh and I don't wish to speak out of turn, but God bears witness to the sins we commit and wants to heal us and for our souls to be set free.

If you find it within you, please start to read about what God can do. He can move mountains.

Do you think he wouldn't help you to overcome your obstacles? Do you think your creator cannot heal your mind? Do you think he isn't powerful enough to take away every single sin you've committed and to make you pure and holy and kind and compassionate and whole again?

He is giving you the option to repent and to learn a new way.

I'm aware a lot of therapists state that there is no cure for cluster B disorders, but God disagrees. Don't play into the fact that you're damned for eternity. YOU CAN CHANGE.

Do the research, become the over-analytical person you hated for discovering and exposing the truth and DO IT FOR YOURSELF. Be the one who can shine a light on how God can heal. How He can do a 180 overnight on your mindset and your personality traits. Throw the masks away. Be who you were created to be. And if you can't do any of this, then please just stop hurting people.

Nobody deserves to be hurt whether for pleasure or retribution.

There is no joy in heartache.

John 16:33
"I have told you these things, so that in me you may have peace. In this world, you will have trouble. But take heart! I have overcome the world."

Empathy

Philippians 2: "Therefore, if you have any encouragement from being united with Christ, if any comfort from his love, if any common sharing in the Spirit, if any tenderness and compassion, then make my joy complete by being like-minded, having the same love, being one in spirit and of one mind. Do nothing out of selfish ambition or vain conceit. Rather, in humility value others above yourselves, not looking to your own interests but each of you to the interests of the others."

One of the most powerful forces on the face of this planet is empathy.

Empathy allows us to feel the joy, pain, love, loss, hurt, wonder and grief of the very essence of life itself.

It makes our hearts skip a beat when we see our children laughing. It makes our eyes fill with tears when we witness someone hurting. It makes our tummies feel warm and fuzzy when we fall in love. It allows us to feel guilty when we know we've hurt someone's feelings. It allows us to extend our sympathies for someone who has lost a loved one. It allows us to put ourselves in someone else's shoes and see things from a different perspective.

Empathy is developed at a very early age, during childhood. Many psychologists and bloggers agree to the fact that one distinguishing factor in personality disorders is the distinct lack or void of empathy.

It is not fully known whether this is a nature or nurture issue. Many argue that when brain scans of those with disorders show no 'lighting up' of their empathetic neurons in a response to stimuli you would expect to get a reaction from, it must be as a result of this part of the brain never having been 'wired right' or activated at the correct point in life.

Others state that as a result of bad parenting, or exposure to narcissistic or emotional abuse, the brain didn't, and won't again have the capacity to develop its empathetic coding.

Although I personally struggle to understand how we can 'teach' someone empathy and acknowledge that a person who enjoys being abusive, narcissistic or diabolically inhuman, is going to agree to access a course to learn how to develop this trait, I do believe that somewhere, in the midst of both these statements, lies a God who can do miracles. You only have to pick up the Bible to see this, but a

google search will also suffice.

There is a father out there who can grow limbs, take away tumours, heal the sick and make the blind see. Do you not believe he can rewire his own creations' neurology any more than he can sew new bones?

Without faith, they say works are dead.

So we the abused, the survivors, the thrivers, need to be empathetic to these people to the point of praying for them, opening up the word of God to them and leading the wolves back to the sheep pen to be healed, but we do not need to give abusers access to our spirit, our psyche and our lives if we intend to look after our own mental emotional and spiritual health.

We need to have faith that only they alone, with their God can do this, but we need to also identify that our empathy can cause us to be caught up playing with the wolves in their own territory, leading us away from our faith and away from our God.

This is the battleground.

Ephesians 6:12

"For we do not wrestle against flesh and blood, but against the rulers, against the authorities, against the cosmic powers over this present darkness, against the spiritual forces of evil in the heavenly places."

Psychology Today (2019) states that empathy is both emotional and cognitive in nature and babies as young as 18 hours old can reflect the emotional expression of those around them. Babies are not taught to do this, it is a fundamental reaction already belonging to them, neurologically speaking their cells are already able to do this. A gift from God? Leading on from this, it is important to note that experiences between these babies and their caregivers are crucial for the nurturing and development of this gift, with associations made between interactions, feelings and rewards. Those babies who are nurtured and parented correctly, who feel safe, secure and loved are more sensitive to others' emotions and needs. This is a fundamental attachment and the quality of such is a predictor of empathy and compassion in later life.

With the rise of mental health conditions and disorders and a broader acceptance of clustered behavioural traits becoming the new normal in this century, it is easy to see how parents are passing down intergenerational curses to their offspring. Being raised by another, who has not taken the time to do the work of self-healing or reflection, can and will raise a generation unable to bear the fruits of the spirit, and thus bring about the end time prophecies mentioned previously, where men are lovers of self, unrighteousness and live to please the ego, not the God of creation.

Compassion and Conscience

1 Peter 3:8: "Be like-minded, be sympathetic, love one another, be compassionate and humble."

1 Kings 2:44: "You know in your heart all the wrong you did."

Another trait linked to abusive personalities is their distinct lack of conscience. Again it is not fully understood how one could not fully feel that actions have consequences, that right and wrong are genuinely two opposite ends of a very sensitive scale, that bad decisions lead to negative outcomes.

It is hard for a neurotypical to comprehend that these people genuinely feel no remorse for the bad things they say and do.

I guess when you feel everything so very deeply, with overflowing empathy, you can't pretend you don't have that emotion any more than a psychopath for example can pretend to feel love. We can all, to a point, put our best act on in order to, for example, impress a potential employer at an interview, but we cannot and do not put on a mask to fool, manipulate and break another person's spirit by pretending to be a person we are not over a longer period of time whilst being aware all the time that you are a liar and a fraud, a con man of the highest regard.

Compassion and conscience clearly do not mix well with personality disorders.

Who could hurt someone (anyone let alone someone you profess to love) by being deceptive and dishonest and spiteful and mean and debasing?

Who could look into someone's eyes and lie to them so easily without a flicker of remorse?

Who could speak to others in a derogatory way and not see them shrink and die a little and not react to their small nuances?

Who could sleep with another person and then come home and say they had been hard at work all day earning money for your 'gifts' (that you never asked for nor wanted in place of real human emotion)?

A narcissist can. A psychopath can. A sociopath can. And they will.

If you don't feel something, it won't bother you. Imagine if your right hand could feel pain but your left hand couldn't. How many of us wouldn't pick up a boiling hot cup of coffee if we were in a rush with our left hand rather than wait until the right hand can tolerate it?

How many personality-disordered people have the want, need or desire to seek help, to change? I'm going to guess at not many. It would almost be akin to a non-personality disordered person wishing to become a narcissist so that they no longer feel the necessity to care about anyone else.

I doubt any of us would choose that path having felt love, compassion, respect and joy – and if it was a choice, imagine how hurt, broken and abused you would need to be in order to become that kind of monster.

There is one particular 'self-confessed' narcissist who frequents YouTube channels on the subject and has written numerous books on the subject who states, as a fact, that he has no plans to change his ways.

He was diagnosed twice with the disorder and has since become what he would coin a 'self-aware' narcissist. He uses this knowledge to spread information about the disorder to the layman, in order that we understand the intricate patterns of their personalities and abusive ways and in order to 'support' (by way of educating) survivors.

This man is extremely self-centred, has no conscience, no empathy and no 'feelings' of love. He will attest to this. He has no desire to learn nor develop these traits either.

Why would he when he doesn't need to? That is the question we need to ask and the answer we feel that we need to understand for our own sanity.

Perhaps, however, the best we can do is to pray for healing, for them and for us and to understand how abusive patterns intergenerationally pass down from father to son / mother to daughter and fundamentally create these dynamics.

Mindfulness and NLP

Romans 12:2: Do not be conformed to this world, but be transformed by the renewal of your mind, that by testing you may discern what is the will of God, what is good and acceptable and perfect.

Colossians 3:2: "Set your minds on things that are above, not on things that are on earth."

1 Timothy 1:7: "For God gave us a spirit not of fear but of power and love and self-control."

2 Cor 10:5: "We demolish arguments and every pretension that set itself against God, and we take captive every thought to make it obedient to Christ."

Philippians 4:8: "Finally brothers, whatever is true, whatever is noble, whatever is pure, whatever is admirable, if anything is excellent and praiseworthy – think about such things."

Many people have recently taken up mindfulness as an exercise by which they can practice the art of grounding. This is a particularly helpful method of controlling the escalating anxiety linked to emotional and psychological abuse. Following my own enlightenment, having been through this kind of abuse throughout my life, I have identified that both mindfulness and NLP are strategies which can help a survivor to focus and overcome intrusive and negative thought patterns associated with trauma.

Having always been an avid learner, and what with the analytical side of my brain wishing to delve deeper into what 'makes me tick', I decided to do an online course in Neurolinguistic Programming, to identify my own patterns of language, thought processing, and unwrap those deep-rooted beliefs I hold about myself and the world around me.

Neuro-Linguistic Programming is how we utilise the language of our mind to achieve specific outcomes. It can be broken down into three chunks;

- Neuro: The mind or neurological wiring, through which experiences are processed by way of our five senses:
  - Vision, Auditory, Kinaesthetic, Olfactory and Gustatory.
- Linguistic: our nonverbal communication systems by which our neural representations are coded, ordered and given meaning, including Pictures, Sounds, Feelings, Tastes, Smells, Words.
- Programming: The ability to learn, understand and adapt the internal programs that we run to achieve specific and desired outcomes.

To understand NLP better, we have to understand that there is cause and effect to all of our behaviours and thought patterns – and then the choices we make because of these.

Cause and Effect

A cause is an event, interaction or process which invites or initiates an effect to take place. For example, the cause of anxiety, as discussed, could be due to the effect of a stimulus such as a trigger to a specific trauma for a certain individual. It could also be something more simple, for example, the cause of my jumping earlier was a loud noise, and the effect was my body reacting to this by alerting me to the potential danger and making me move suddenly, and somewhat unconsciously as my body had no time to process it – but the neural pathways in my mind already had.

This unconscious space, or what NLP labelled 'the comfort zone', is where we spend most of our time, the space where we are neither at cause nor effect and we are just in a state of 'being'. Or perhaps, I could argue, within the peace that God promised. Our minds are after all made of matter, a part of our cellular composition, our flesh and bones, but as we know we only use approximately 10% of our brains, and the other 90% is a mystery. Is it in this space, this black hole known only to God, still unknown to science, that we have a relationship with God? With the universe and the unknown? Where dreams and visions arise?

Cause and effect and the comfort zone may be more related than we think, with our objectivity of each individual situation. Sometimes we may feel neither cause nor effect however if we change our perceptions or thought processes, we can become a greater force of cause for our own life's outcomes.

The cause-and-effect exercise in my training course highlighted the fact that even though things may appear out of my control, or to be 'happening to me' (effect), I was indeed in a position to highlight how I could change my mindset and become the cause for most of the things I listed. It is a shift in perspective and accountability to become the cause of your own life's actions.

Scientifically, we all have internal processors or maps that can be 'rewritten' or 'rewired' in order to change our perceptions or processing of information and, thus, our own patterns of behaviour, through NLP, EMDR, CBT and other psychological theories. Spiritually, we can ask for more. God can do miracles. Personally, I believe this understanding is the foundation stone for overcoming many barriers to achieving success in areas of trauma, triggers, and internal self-doubt.

NLP training made me realise that people act or behave from the place of their own understanding of the world around them, their past experiences and their own ability to process information. People can often project their own 'identity' or beliefs/behaviours onto others as that's how they see and deal with the world internally.

When I feel the 'effect' of someone else's behaviour, that it is in fact just their internal process that I am reacting to, and not necessarily the situation as a whole.

I still find it somewhat interesting that the mind doesn't process negatives, and this highlights the importance of positive affirmations, creating a new map of outcomes just by using the relevant language that the mind understands and can adapt and react to. This is something we can do individually and with others whilst interacting to change the cause and effect of all of our interactions, in friendship, in work and in relationships.

How can we positively apply this knowledge, these techniques and these skills in our lives, in our work, and in order to help other people?

To become more mindful and accountable of the words we use, the thought processes we allow to develop and the effect of what we 'take on' in life allows us to reflect on situations and circumstances to see where and how we have been the cause or have been at the effect of our own being, and therefore allows us to change our relationship with self and others. In my workplace, for example, as a nurse, I can relate this to the biopsychosocial model of psychology to help me to provide better outcomes for those using the service. Holistic care is something that is considered gold-standard across the world, as to treat a disease you have to treat the whole person, and to me, this means their body, their mind, their heart, their hurts and their soul. Any of these that are out of balance will have an impact on all of the other elements. 'The body keeps the score' is not only a powerful psychological book but an entirely true concept in physical and mental health care.

There is clearly a correlation between internal representations and mental health and well-being. The mind is a powerful tool and learning how to deconstruct information and 'reprocess' it will improve the state of mind and body. By supporting the brain's ability to process information (positively!) and by consciously becoming the 'cause' of our own destiny, there will be an automatic shift whereby the mind will react to the newly constructed neuro pathways and become more able and positive.

This begins, one could suggest, by accepting that we live, in part at least, through that unconscious part of the mind. Where perhaps that spirit abides.

The prime responsibilities or functions of the unconscious mind are to store and organise our memories, process our emotions, repress negative memories and emotions (perhaps for protection), and keep a blueprint of the body now and of how it could be in a perfect health state (higher state of consciousness), preserve the body, control and maintain perceptions regularly and telepathically, maintain and generate habits.

Therefore, the unconscious requires repetition of something, to develop or create a new habit.

The Bible reinforces this notion, and as a Christian, meditation and prayer are interchangeable notions. Prayer is a structured way to reflect upon God, via the neuro, linguistic route, in order to programme our minds to seek the revelations of the creator. The Holy Ghost?

Deliberately focusing on specific thoughts, better understanding their meaning and encompassing the relationship between yourself and the promises of God, in the word (Bible) can create a new habit, helping you to see yourself as the son, or daughter of God through love, acceptance and wholeness. What is more interesting is that research has shown those whom have faith in God tend to heal or deal with traumas quicker and at a higher level than those without faith.

There are many scriptures that lead us to prayer; to spend time in direct mindful correspondence with the Lord.

Psalm 65:2

"For God alone, O my soul, wait in silence, for my hope is from him."

Psalm 84:1–2

"How lovely is your dwelling place, O Lord of hosts! My soul longs, yes, faints for the courts of the Lord; my heart and flesh sing for joy to the living God."

Thessalonians 5:16–18

"Rejoice always, pray without ceasing, give thanks in all circumstances; for this is the will of God in Christ Jesus for you."

James 5:13

"Is anyone among you in trouble? Let them pray. Is anyone happy? Let them sing songs of praise."

And if we look at the life of Jesus, the son of God, we can see why prayer is important. The word 'prayer' is used alongside Jesus countless times in scripture, and was performed before many of his works; prior to his baptism, prior to evangelism, prior to choosing his disciples prior to his death. Before important occurrences in his life. Jesus also prayed after these occurrences, to renew his spirit and, perhaps, to renew his unconscious (soul) mind and realign his physical (neurological pathways) with God.

Mark 11:24

Therefore I tell you, whatever you ask for in prayer, believe that you have received it, and it will be yours.

NLP identifies that an individual can enter what is known as a 'learning state', whereby we can focus on one particular area (e.g. a spot on a plain wall) but shift our perceptions to expand our focus. Upon entering the learning state, a sense of calmness and an understanding that although focusing on one area, we can expand our field of perception and therefore process more information than we expect ensues. It allows us to think 'outside the box' about what else was happening around us, rather than 'to us', therefore allowing conscious acknowledgement that there is more information being processed by our unconscious, than what we are initially aware of.

In a separate psychological model, four stages of learning competence are considered as a 'conscious competence' model, relating to the psychological states involved in the process of progressing from incompetence to competence in any given skill, or effect relating to a cause. People may have several set effects (behavioural patterns), and each will typically be at one of the stages of the model at a given time. Many effects/behaviours require practice to remain at a high level of competence, or the 'correct' response to a trigger.

The four stages of learning about this unconscious incompetence mean:

1) That we don't know what we don't know, or we have no idea how or what to learn, what I am good or bad at or what behaviours in me are less than ideal, or can harm or trigger others.
2) Conscious incompetence makes us aware that we are not very good at something. That our thought patterns harm us, make us feel 'less than' or hurt others.

3) Conscious competence means that I can do something but I need to be aware and concentrated to achieve it. I need to acknowledge why I'm acting the way I do, reacting the way I do, and what I can do to change it.
4) Unconscious competence, which means I have no awareness of my ability to achieve something. This is where we need to ponder the notion that we learn through nurture and nature and as we ask to be made more self-aware, we are given knowledge by way of relationships with others and by God.

The habits developed work through these stages in order, however working backwards can rewire and reconstruct our learned behaviour or patterns by breaking things down and improving our competence. If we again reflect on this within our own professions, we can see how we develop skills that are now unconsciously competent (i.e. we can do them without much thought) but if we go back to being consciously competent then we may see from a different angle how we could improve our skills and therefore provide a better service or outcome for ourselves and our peers/partners/families.

The psychological, scientific approach and model outlined is a skill which can be used in all areas of life to break down patterns of behaviour and to reprogramme or rewire the brain (and set actions) in order to achieve more focused outcomes. I believe that by using this process in my work and everyday life, I have become more aware of my own actions and how these can lead to positive change. I can also see how the veil between science and God is thin and how it is impossible to believe one exists without the other.

Timothy 3:16

"All Scripture is breathed out by God and profitable for teaching, for reproof, for correction, and for training in righteousness."

Proverbs 1:5

"Let the wise hear and increase in learning, and the one who understands obtain guidance."

Romans 15:4

"For whatever was written in former days was written for our instruction, that through endurance and through the encouragement of the Scriptures we might have hope."

I've personally found that it is much more natural for me to take the path of wanting to learn and achieve more. It is unnatural for me personally to dwell on the negative path, however, I can see that it is a choice in how I allow my mind to act and interact with my surroundings and my stimuli.

It has to be a conscious choice to find these situations, processes and skills in order to think outside the box and rewire the narrative the world wishes to teach you, and achieve more.

This is where curiosity kicks in and I begin to develop an acute awareness of the fact that we sometimes don't see the obvious because our minds are wired to only process what we already know (our unconscious programming from our lived experiences). This highlights the structured way that we adapt due to our own internal processes and that, with conscious thought, we are able to deconstruct any limiting factors to learn or develop better skills and coping mechanisms.

I believe that by becoming aware of this functioning pattern, I am now able to use this in my prayerful life and meditation practice, and any future endeavour by understanding that there is always more that I don't know, and I can be curious enough to go out and learn it or that if I am unconsciously doing something, that I can work my way backwards to ensure I am indeed doing it to the best of my ability and not just relying on old patterns which have become ingrained in my mind.

We have to want to become better people to have impactful change for ourselves and those we share our lives with.

Present vs Preoccupied

Luke 9:62: "No procrastination. No backward looks. You can't put God's kingdom off till tomorrow. Seize the day."

Matthew 11:28–30: "Come to Me, all you who labour and are heavy laden, and I will give you rest. Take My yoke upon you and learn from Me, for I am gentle and lowly in heart, and you will find rest for your souls. For My yoke is easy and My burden is light."

John 14:27: "Peace I leave with you, My peace I give to you; not as the world gives do I give to you. Let not your heart be troubled, neither let it be afraid."

One element of NLP is techniques that have been developed to change negative thought processes. I would encourage anybody that is interested in the scientific elements of neurological wiring to look more closely into this, as I won't be elaborating on these techniques within this book. My intention to mention it here is to allow the reader to make correlations between what NLP is aiming to achieve, and how the Word of God and faith in Jesus can lead to the same outcome. I guess as I've already alluded to, it is a science entwined with religious fact, rather than a Versus connotation.

Throughout my life, I always held a limited belief that I was not good enough (as a person) or had nothing to offer to someone else (in terms of employment and relationships). I now KNOW, realistically, this isn't true, however, it still affects how I limit myself.

With the realisation through NLP that I learn and interact more within an audial-digital environment, I can see how I've come to this conclusion mostly via self-talk (and thus, self-analysis as discussed previously).

It's still difficult to do some days, but through my faith in the Word of God, I can see that he has changed me from that girl who wasn't good enough, to one who uses gratitude, love and self-respect to reflect every success and victory the Lord has bestowed upon me. The change in my thought pattern comes as a direct result of not listening to the world, but to the Word.

Being present is something that I have had to learn, but something that I absolutely attempt to live by. When we are present, we automatically switch off those negative thought processes, and it also brings peace.

When we are present, in the moment and there is no cause and no effect, we live in that unconscious state, the part of the brain that is unknown, the presence of God.

There is no trigger, no trauma, no past, no future. Just us and our creator breathing in peace and stillness and quiet and breathing out worry and anxiety and stressors.

It is in these moments of aloneness that we can feel the most content.

For me, that looks like the ability to appreciate and have gratitude for every single second. I am able to see the true beauty of life itself. Every breath is a promise from God, every cell in the matrix of my body and mind whole and complete and working just as He said. The blood pumping his word through my veins, encouraging my muscles, my heart, to continue beating. My eyes take in my present surroundings and there is no history in them except that of him, the grass and the trees and the fields and the sun and moon and stars. There is perfection in every single thing. A perfection we cannot appreciate in preoccupation.

The world today is made up of distractions. Distractions to God's word, to our ability to be alone, to our ability to grow. Principalities of darkness are now accepted and impose on our ability to be present, with ourselves or in relationship with others.

Social media has created a platform where we are more concerned about other people's 'happy lives' than our own mental health. A community of people who all wish to look the same or idolise the behaviours so closely related to the clustered disorders mentioned. Where wickedness is on the tongue or envy is completely accepted as the norm. People celebrate being lost and having no self-identity as if it is progression. Mental health is a public health crisis and yet we sit back and allow this to continue under a democracy run by liars and thieves and people who would rather have a fast buck in the bank than a humble and giving spirit. The corruption is accepted by the masses who are following man rather than God.

I've had close friends who have been so troubled by society recently, so troubled by the news and social media that they have become so downcast, rendering themselves susceptible to depression and yet nobody dares speak out about its cause – the effect is the depression – the cause, sin.

The Bible reminds us that the devil is a liar. Why do you think that society is crumbling? Instead of accepting God and peace, people accept what society has made acceptable, lies and destruction and deception and business of mind. If we cannot live in peace, we live in cause and effect, and out of the unconscious space where we find peace, in God's presence.

2 Corinthians 11:3

"But I am afraid that as the serpent deceived Eve by his cunning, your thoughts will be led astray from a sincere and pure devotion to Christ."

John 8:44

"You are of your father the devil, and your will is to do your father's desires. He was a murderer from the beginning and has nothing to do with the truth because there is no truth in him. When he lies, he speaks out of his own character, for he is a liar and the father of lies."

Romans 14:19

"So then let us pursue what makes for peace and for mutual upbuilding."

John 16:33

"I have said these things to you, that in me you may have peace. In the world, you will have tribulation. But take heart; I have overcome the world."

Philippians 4:7

"And the peace of God, which surpasses all understanding, will guard your hearts and your minds in Christ Jesus."

Finding Your Purpose

Philippians 2:1–8: "If then there is any encouragement in Christ, any consolation from love, any sharing in the Spirit, any compassion and sympathy, make my joy complete: be of the same mind, having the same love, being in full accord and of one mind. Do nothing from selfish ambition or conceit but in humility regard others as better than yourselves. Let each of you look not to your own interests, but to the interests of others. Let the same mind be in you that was in Christ Jesus, who, though he was in the form of God, did not regard equality with God as something to be exploited, but emptied himself, taking the form of a slave, being born in human likeness. And being found in human form, he humbled himself and became obedient to the point of death – even death on a cross."

Day on day, week on week, year on year, we all navigate through times and seasons. The Bible says that there is a time and a purpose for everything under heaven.

Ecclesiastes 3: 1–8

To everything there is a season and a time to every purpose under the heaven:

A time to be born, and a time to die; a time to plant, and a time to pluck up that which is planted; a time to kill, and a time to heal; a time to break down, and a time to build up; a time to weep, and a time to laugh; a time to mourn, and a time to dance; a time to cast away stones, and a time to gather stones together; a time to embrace, and a time to refrain from embracing; a time to get, and a time to lose; a time to keep, and a time to cast away; a time to rend, and a time to sew; a time to keep silence, and a time to speak; a time to love, and a time to hate; a time of war, and a time of peace.

If we take this as a blueprint; we could all relate to the fact that our lives have a purpose and a plan, set out before we were even conceived.

Jeremiah 1:5

"Before I formed you in the womb, I knew you, before you were born, I set you apart; I appointed you as a prophet to the nations."

In that respect, all we have to do is focus on the fact that God is the creator of all, He is in control and each step on our journey not only belongs to Him but is ordained by Him. The purpose for us is to find that place of awakening where we fully comprehend that nothing is an accident, nothing is by chance, and nothing is impossible for the sons and daughters of the creator.

Job is a prime example of this; a man who was so consumed by his faith and love for God, that every attack and trial of the enemy set forth upon him was thwarted. Job never gave up hope, and called out to God in his suffering;

Job 42: 2

I know that You can do all things and that no plan of Yours can be thwarted.

If we think in terms of traumas, trials and mental health, it is easy to understand how people can become so downtrodden and angry. It is easy to see how trials and tribulations, injustices and attacks can change a person's mindset and make them play out traits associated with that level of hurt and pain. But God has called us to do better.

We are not what has hurt us, we are spiritual beings, living out an eternal battle between good and bad, joy and pain, hate and suffering. The choices we make are all ours to own. We can choose to be a victim of our pain and suffering in this world, or we can choose to lay all our hurt and suffering at his feet and to learn and understand that these trials are just a part of the bigger picture and can shape us into a person who has character, integrity and righteousness as our foundation.

Romans 8:28

"And we know that for those who love God all things work together for good, for those who are called according to His purpose."

John 16:33

"I have said these things to you, that in me you may have peace. In the world, you will have tribulation. But take heart; I have overcome the world."

Ephesians 6: 10–18

Finally, be strong in the Lord and in His mighty power. Put on the full armour of God, so that you can take your stand against the devil's schemes. For our struggle is not against flesh and blood, but against the rulers, against the authorities, against the powers of this dark world and against the spiritual forces of evil in the heavenly realms. Therefore put on the full armour of God, so that when the day of evil comes, you may be able to stand your ground, and after you have done everything, to stand. Stand firm then, with the belt of truth buckled around your waist, with the breastplate of righteousness in place, and with your feet fitted with the readiness that comes from the gospel of peace. In addition to all this, take up the shield of faith, with which you can extinguish all the flaming arrows of the evil one. Take the helmet of salvation and the sword of the Spirit, which is the word of God. And pray in the Spirit on all occasions with all kinds of prayers and requests. With this in mind, be alert and always keep on praying for all the Lord's people.

Prayers that Break Chains

Psalm 107:10–14
"Some sat in darkness and in the shadow of death, prisoners in affliction and in irons, for they had rebelled against the words of God, and spurned the counsel of the most High. So He bowed their hearts down with hard labour; they fell down, with none to help. Then they cried to the Lord in their trouble, and He delivered them from their distress. He brought them out of darkness and the shadow of death and burst their bonds apart."

We want to ask God to break the bonds of trauma, to rid the psyche of self-blame, shame, guilt and hurt, and to ensure our wounds are healed so that they can no longer be penetrated by dark souls seeking a target like a heat-seeking missile. It is well known in the cycle of abuse that abusers look for victims with 'issues', or past hurts that aren't healed. The cycle they use disorientates, confuses, manipulates and aims to gain control. The love bombing and infatuation result in the release of highly addictive chemicals in the target's bloodstream, adrenaline, cortisol, feel good factors. Like nicotine, the victim becomes reliant on getting that 'hit' and will continue to seek this out, even at the expense of suffering devaluation and pushing boundaries. We reason with ourselves that the person isn't truly abusive, the 'real' them is the person we first met, who adored and cherished us, put us on a pedestal and made us feel 'set apart' and loved. We negate the abuse and focus on the good. What we need to pray for, and get deliverance from, is our own lack of self-love and self-esteem. An abusive entity will delve deep into your own lack of self-worth, find your vulnerabilities, and play these off against you. The resulting cycle will see you diminish and lose hope in anyone outside of your abusive situation.

The key to this is to ask God to come into your life, to remember who you are and to lose the chains that bind you.

Psalm 107:14

"He brought them out of darkness and the shadow of death And broke their bands apart."

Nahum 1:13

"So now, I will break his yoke bar from upon you, And I will tear off your shackles."

Psalm 2:3

"Let us tear their fetters apart and cast away their cords from us!"

Psalm 107:16

"For He has shattered gates of bronze and cut bars of iron asunder."

Psalm 107:10

"There were those who dwelt in darkness and in the shadow of death, prisoners in misery and chains."

Isaiah 58:6

"Is this not the fast which I choose, To loosen the bonds of wickedness, To undo the bands of the yoke, And to let the oppressed go free And break every yoke?"

Jeremiah 30:8

'It shall come about on that day,' declares the Lord of hosts, 'that I will break his yoke from off their neck and will tear off their bonds; and strangers will no longer make them their slaves.

Isaiah 10:27

"So it will be in that day, that his burden will be removed from your shoulders and his yoke from your neck, and the yoke will be broken because of fatness."

Jeremiah 5:5

"I will go to the great And will speak to them, For they know the way of the Lord And the ordinance of their God." But they too, with one accord, have broken the yoke And burst the bonds.

Mark 5:4

Because he had often been bound with shackles and chains, and the chains had been torn apart by him and the shackles broken in pieces, and no one was strong enough to subdue him.

There are many verses in the bible about breaking chains and living freely. God has not given us a spirit of fear and loathing and self-hate. He has given us life and life eternal. We are not here to suffer, we are here to grow closer to him as righteous spirits in faith, hope and love. These prayer points are powerful as we can decree and declare that this is our portion. We can cast off the work of the enemy and accept the all-encompassing love of the saviour. It is our voice, our choice. Choose your next season. Choose the Word.

Conclusion

12. 1 Peter 3:3–4

"Don't be concerned about the outward beauty of fancy hairstyles, expensive jewellery, or beautiful clothes. You should clothe yourselves instead with the beauty that comes from within, the unfading beauty of a gentle and quiet spirit, which is so precious to God."

It has taken many years, new experiences and toing and froing between the self and my God to finish this book. I still struggle some days with living out the knowledge, research and faith found within these chapters, and life still continues to offer curve-balls interacting with the dynamics of others and with the true self of me. I write this conclusion at a time when I am experiencing a new trauma within a close familial relationship and whilst it has been challenging, I am learning to accept that life was never meant to be easy. It is, however, supposed to be peaceful and lived in the light of God. One of the fruits of the spirit is peace, and never in my life have I experienced such profound peace as when God called me home and awakened me to this knowledge and profound love. I enjoy being alone almost as much as being part of a congregation of others who are now my extended family. Melody and I, over the last eight years have had many instances of what we consider supernatural alignments within our personal and spiritual lives and have discussed the topics in these books to a place where I've finally found the courage to publish them. It was serendipity, or an act of God that day to change our stars and hopefully, yours too.

We all have times and seasons and we all make mistakes and live life imperfectly, but God is there through it all.

In every serendipity, in every interaction, in every sense he gave us ears to hear, eyes to see and a heart to love. The mind is where it begins and ends, in its perfect peace.

Pray for each other, set boundaries to protect your heart and be kind. Trust that God is always working in your life, even when times are difficult, and he will give you, his promise. He will break every chain that binds you and wrap you in his eternal love and grace because you, daughter and son, are so, so precious and faultless to God.

Amen.

References

Anxiety and Depression Association of America (ADAA) (2016) What is Anxiety and Depression. Available from: *https://adaa.org/understanding-anxiety* (Accessed 14/08/2022).

Burgees, L (2018) What are Personality Disorders. Medical News Today (Online) Available from: *https://www.medicalnewstoday.com/articles/320508.php* (Accessed: 10/05/2018).

Gorman. J, M. (1996) Comorbid depression and anxiety spectrum disorders. Available from: *https://pubmed.ncbi.nlm.nih.gov/9166648/* (Accessed: 14/08/2022).

Mentalhelp.net (2016) DSM-5: The Ten Personality Disorders: Cluster B (online) Available from: *https://www.mentalhelp.net/articles/dsm-5-the-ten-personality-disorders-cluster-b/* (Accessed: 10/05/2018).

Psychology Today (2019) How Children Develop Empathy. Empathy is a work-in-progress throughout childhood and adolescence. Available from:
https://www.psychologytoday.com/gb/blog/smart-parenting-smarter-kids/201905/how-children-develop-empathy
(Accessed: 14/08/2022).

The Mental Health Foundation (2017) UK and World-wide Mental Health Statistics. Available at:
https://www.mentalhealth.org.uk/explore-mental-health/statistics/uk-worldwide-statistics
(Accessed 14/08/2022).

Women's Aid (2016) Domestic Abuse and Your Mental Health. Available from:
https://www.womensaid.org.uk/information-support/the-survivors-handbook/domestic-abuse-and-your-mental-health/
(Accessed 14/08/2022).